THE PROSTATE STORM

One Guy Battles Prostate Cancer,
BPH and Prostatitis, and Bets on a Cure-All

Steve Vogel

First Edition January 2011
Second Edition June 2011
Printed in the United States of America
Published by Red Willow Publishing
Book cover and design by Lorraine Vogel

ISBN-10 1936539012
ISBN-13 9781936539017

DISCLAIMER
This book is written as a source of information only. The information contained in this book is by no means considered a substitute for the advice of a qualified medical professional, who should always be consulted before beginning any new diet or other health program. All efforts have been made to ensure the accuracy of the information in this book as of the date published. The author expressly disclaims responsibility for any adverse effects arising from the use or application of the information contained therein.

For my son, Nick, brother, Kurt, and nephews, Kurt Jr., Michael, Matt and Zack, all of whom share a family history of prostates run amok.

Endless thanks to my wife, Lorraine, for encouraging me to turn prostate cancer into this book, and for just being there through all the twists and turns of both.

> *"**Prostate cancer** is always found together with **prostatitis** and all men will probably get both diseases if they live long enough ... Both conditions are currently at epidemic, if not pandemic, levels."*
>
> ~ Ronald E. Wheeler, M.D.
> Medical Director of the Prostatitis
> and Prostate Cancer Center

> *I hit the prostate trifecta with my biopsy report yesterday. Prostatitis. BPH. Prostate cancer. I leak, I burn, I go often and at all hours. The plumbing is broken. I am the guy in the TV commercial, peeing while my friends raft and bike and golf and ski... and now I am one of those unlucky one-of-every-six guys diagnosed with prostate cancer. My gut tells me this has been building for years – but what's the connection between these diseases? My mainstream doctors say "None" or "Not enough science"... my alternative doc says "they're all linked."*
> *So what's the the truth?*
>
> ~ From my personal notes, a day after my diagnosis

TABLE OF CONTENTS

Introduction
A PROSTATE RUN AMOK

Hello, my name is Steve and I dribble in my pants ...

That was the confessional first line of a blog I started writing days after being diagnosed with prostate cancer. The information in this book spilled out of my whole cancer experience, from the pre-diagnosis inconvenient leaking and chronic urinary tract infections ... to my emotional awakening as a newbie cancer host ... to the aftershocks of treatment ... to learning what doctors *don't* tell you ... to discovering my incredible ignorance about the walnut-sized gland (growing into a small apple) that I had sat on for 55 years. My prostate.

I'm not a doctor or a medical expert, by any stretch. I'm a prostate cancer survivor, with a background as a freelance writer, researcher and journalist. I'm writing not to persuade anyone to ascribe to a specific lifestyle, try some off-the-wall cancer cure, or see a certain kind of doctor.

If anything, I would recommend consulting with as many experts as you can (mainstream and alternative) *and* consider all points of view regarding the prostate and its health. Why? Because *no one* can advise with absolute certainty on what you should do or not do, take or not take. Treatment options, even prostate cancer screening, are all subjects of stormy controversy in an oftentimes bewildering prostate world.

My intent in telling my story is to share what I came to

learn about prostate disease and, if you're a sufferer, to help you on your journey to better health.

An otherwise healthy and active guy, I ran to stay fit for 30 years, including running 13 marathons from New York to Chicago to Boston. During that time, I paid no attention whatsoever to my prostate, nor to the clues that trouble was brewing below my belt.

My prostate took a turn south around age 47, about the time my family doctor first performed a digital rectal exam on me. As I pulled up my pants, he snapped off his glove and told me my prostate was moderately enlarged. Weary of what that meant, I asked if there was anything I could do about it. He called my enlarged prostate "just a sign of aging" and told me "not to worry." Then he recommended I take an annual PSA test for cancer as a precautionary measure — but he didn't suggest anything else. That was it. So I followed my doctor's instructions. I didn't worry about it. I did nothing else.

Big mistake.

Over the next eight years, my urinary issues went downhill at an accelerating clip. What started out as annoyances and inconveniences, like extra trips to the bathroom, became all-consuming. When my misery meter finally redlined, I had to urinate 10 to 20 times day and night. Urinary tract infections became somewhat frequent. Sex burned like I was ejaculating the tiniest of razor blades.

On many occasions while running, I peed blood. The first time it happened, I was nearing the pagodas of

Chinatown, just past the 21-mile mark of the Chicago marathon. Before getting into the big crowds, I stopped to take a leak … and out came a cup full of hot burgundy-hued urine. I freaked.

It was the first time I'd seen so much blood in my urine, but not the last. At marathons and half-marathons in Tampa, Palm Beach, Miami, New York, and again in Chicago — not to mention on too many training runs to count — a burning sensation would send me off into the weeds or a port-o-potty, only to observe the red urine stream coming out of me. Or, there would be the burning and overwhelming urgency to go, but nothing except maybe a drop or two, was there.

I got used to it on my long runs. My doctors thought it might be something called jogger's hematuria, a common phenomena among long distance runners. But I wasn't sure. Sometimes a urine test revealed an infection, sometimes not. To me, it all seemed connected with my assorted plumbing problems.

Unfortunately, no one had any answers. And it just got worse.

For the most part, I lived with all of these annoyances and discomforts. I learned to adapt.

Take the dribbling, for instance. It got terribly embarrassing to me, especially during my son's junior season playing high school baseball. That's when I started to wear untucked shirts with long tails at his games. I would have to go to the bathroom so often, I wanted to hide the inevitable dribbling that might soak through the crotch of my pants. If I wore khakis, it stayed wet until it dried yellow.

Can you imagine? I was a former coach myself, an active father in the baseball program, never missed a game … *I'm my kid's dad* … and I couldn't stop the dribbling in my drawers. It got so bad, one day I found myself shopping in Walgreen's for diapers. That's what happens when a sick, faltering, neglected prostate goes completely haywire. In the meantime, my urologist's sage counsel — "It's a natural part aging, not to worry" — kept repeating in my head.

Really? This is natural? This is pathetic.

The worst part, however, was the reoccurring bouts with acute bladder and urinary tract infections, which were always treated with rounds of antibiotics. The infections brought on fever and chills and burning urination. They came on so frequently and severely that the old drugs I took no longer worked. I needed more powerful antibiotics to find relief.

One day my prostate and urinary tract became so swollen and inflamed with infection, it squeezed my urethra shut and prevented me from peeing altogether.

So even the annoying dribbling stopped.

I know what it feels like to give birth to craggy kidney stones. But a *closed urethra* that dammed up 800 milliliters of urine (when the normal full bladder holds maybe 300 milliliters) fits into a pain category all by itself. I ended up in a local hospital emergency room where doctors had to open a passageway with a catheter, threaded up my penis all the way to the bladder — finally bursting open the dam. Trust me, you want to pass on that experience.

The problem at the time, and the problem my doctors consistently misdiagnosed, was chronic and acute prostatitis, which spawned infections that climbed into my bladder. Misdiagnosing this problem is not uncommon, and neither is one condition leading to another. I've since found out that many researchers believe that chronic and persistent prostatitis, by definition a disease of inflammation, may actually lead to prostate cancer.

In the aftermath of my urgent trip to the hospital for the catheter, I consulted several doctors, including a second urologist, all of whom told me there was not much they could do to help me "cure" what had become a chronic condition. Being stupid about all things prostate, I was shocked that mainstream doctors could do little more than simply treat these symptoms. These were common diseases, after all, that had been around forever. While stronger antibiotics seemed to mercifully knock out the infections and inflammation for me, I wanted to *solve* my problem *without drugs* and to get to the root cause, not just find temporary relief.

So I did something I should've done years earlier: I consulted an alternative medicine practitioner-slash-acupuncturist who introduced me to herbal remedies, organic teas, colon cleanses, dietary changes and acupuncture needles. That first day as I whined on about my prostate miseries, he said the magic word — he promised me a "cure."

Skeptical, I nonetheless followed this doctor's advice to

the letter. I gobbled down a concoction of herbs, antioxidants, high concentrate beta-sitosterol and nettle root. I reduced the fats and simple sugars in my diet. I tried a few sessions of acupuncture and even did a lightweight colon cleanse.

And guess what? A couple months passed, and my urinary problems started to recede en masse. It was incredible. I slept through most nights again without peeing. Even the inconvenient dribble became hardly worth mentioning.

Alas, too little, too late. Just as my prostate seemed to take a turn for the better, I took my annual PSA test for prostate cancer. That was in December of 2007.

The results came back with an alarming spike in my PSA level, indicating it might be prostate cancer, but it might also be another infection ... or the level simply could have been inflated by having sex or taking a bike ride the day before.

The PSA test, I learned, is *not* very reliable. But I took it again a week later and got the same result of 6.6 ng/ml — nanograms per milliliter of blood. Not a huge number as PSAs go, but it had spiked up from a baseline of 1 ng/ml a year earlier — and that sudden jump was alarming.

To rule out infection, my doctor put me on more high-powered antibiotics for six weeks. But my third PSA level also came back significantly elevated at 5.6 ng/ml. Again, not off the charts, but because it had risen more than a couple points within one year, and stayed up, meant the doctor had to recommend a biopsy. A biopsy, not a PSA test, establishes the presence of prostate cancer.

Sure enough, the biopsy found microbits of cancer, speckled in two tiny clusters along the outer rim of my prostate. The pathology report also revealed a prostate swollen to the brim with prostatitis (inflammation) and benign prostate hyperplasia (the enlarged prostate).

I had hit the jackpot — the prostate triple-whammy.

If that weren't sobering enough, only days later an ultrasound on a strange black protrusion behind my knee revealed I had an eight-inch-long blood clot in my calf, a deep vein thrombosis, or DVT, *likely caused by the cancer*. But unlike the cancer, the clot threatened to kill me, not years from now, but *NOW*. Should a chunk of the clot break off and migrate to my lung, I faced having a pulmonary embolism.

This was plainly a lousy week.

Could any of the problems with my prostate — the BPH, the chronic and acute prostatitis, the urinary tract and bladder infections, the prostate cancer, and by extension, the DVT — been avoided? What if I'd taken better care of my prostate much earlier, like eight years earlier when my doctor first told me my prostate was mildly enlarged and not to worry?

Should I have worried even a little? Or done something like eat more fruits and veggies? Or not consumed ibuprofen like jelly beans for my running aches and pains? Or done more colon cleanses? Or learned how to perform prostate massages on myself? Or downed more saw palmetto with a cocktail of anti-inflammatory antioxidants?

What could I have done — if anything?

Which brings me to writing this book.

The Prostate Storm includes my story about a prostate run amok, the cancer diagnosis, treatment and aftermath — that's Part 1 and Part 5. The interior Parts 2, 3 and 4 include new research and good-things-every-guy-should-know that I discovered during and after my prostate cancer treatment.

As I wrote in my blog (www.theprostatestorm.blogspot. com), I wish I would have had this book to read years ago. If I had known even half of the information in this book when my prostate issues began, I would've been able to nurture a healthier prostate before things slid off into the ditch.

The title of the book refers to several "storms" swirling around the prostate. There are, in a sense, perfect storms of controversy surrounding PSA screening, overtreatment issues, perplexing therapy choices weighed against potentially devastating side effects, and the emerging role of diet and inflammation as triggers for prostate cancer.

The Prostate Storm theme is also a pretty fair analogy for how it all feels, physically and emotionally, when a prostate progressively falters — from those early waves of annoyance and inconvenience, to bigger frontal systems of discomfort and pain, and finally to those high-pressure nor'easters of fear and dread.

Throughout this book, I cut through the medical clutter the best I could — or at least make the information more easily digestible to all of us who don't hold medical degrees. And because even cancer can be funny, I hope there's a grin or two for you as well.

From prostatitis and BPH to cancer, the prostate in

American men is under siege by diet and genetics and advancing age. Some factors we can't control; others we definitely can. Still, it's safe to say that most men don't know what's sneaking up on them, much less what to do about it.

Today, 1 out of every 5 or 6 American men will be diagnosed with prostate cancer — yet nearly all men will eventually have it if they live long enough. That's right — almost 100 percent. Our prostates breed cancer, though not everyone needs to be treated with expensive and aggressive therapies. About half of all prostate cancer is a low-grade, nonlethal variety that a guy can live with as a chronic and often asymptomatic condition. The other types can be extremely aggressive and even resistant to treatment — potentially very dangerous. Sorting out which is lethal and which isn't is what the best scientists are now trying to figure out.

If you're reading this book because you've been recently diagnosed with prostate cancer, I urge you not to panic. A cancer diagnosis can be a frightening and confusing experience, but time is on your side to make the right treatment decision for you.

Prostate cancer tends to grow very slowly. Its cure rate is the highest among all cancers, especially if it's caught early. So slow down, get multiple expert opinions, learn as much as you can, and keep an open mind. You don't want to make a decision in haste that you'll regret later.

For the rest of you, get tested annually. When to start and when to stop is a matter of much debate, even among the experts. Generally, at age 75, prostate cancer may be so slow growing, it's no longer life threatening, so the screen is not as useful as it was earlier in life. Younger men, however, should start testing as early as age 40, especially if you have a history of prostate cancer in the family.

The science no one argues with is that if you can identify most types of prostate cancer early with a PSA screen, the odds are excellent — virtually 100 percent — you will die of something else.

Which is everyone's goal. LOL.

Best of luck and good reading,

Steve

Postscript: This is the second edition of *The Prostate Storm*. Along with updating content and citing new studies, I added a new last chapter, a stark reminder (at least for me), that prostate cancer isn't something you treat and move on from, but a journey. Aptly, a marathon.

> ▶ Blog: April 4, 2008
> Every morning this first week (after the diagnosis), it's the same thing over and over again...I crawl out of bed at 3 a.m. to take a leak, and just as I get to the can, I hear the same words pop in my head, "Hey Dude, you have prostate cancer!... as if to say, You're screwed now!" Talk about a morning jolt. My subconscious must be processing this new reality for me. But I just feel like a spectator, no longer in charge...

Part 1

MY STORY COULD BE ANYONE'S

Diagnosis Day: Full Fear Ahead

The day of my diagnosis for prostate cancer, I sat alone in a small, windowless exam room, waiting for my results, staring at a cracked plastic model of a penile implant. Talk about a bad omen. After a good fifteen minutes, my urologist, Dr. WS, finally makes his appearance, shakes my hand loosely and leans back against the wall to discuss the results of my biopsy.

As he starts to speak, he suddenly drops his eyes, which I find a bit disturbing because he had no notes or file in hand. How many times has he avoided eye contact with a patient and looked to the floor while delivering good news about cancer? C'mon. No eye to eye, the broken penis — all bad signs. I could feel this wasn't going to go well.

Finally: I'm sorry, he tells me, your biopsy came back positive. You have prostate cancer.

Whack, there it is, the words floating out loud, filling the little room. I go totally blank. I feel nothing. Not a sickening panic in my gut. No gripping fear. My urologist had just dropped the bomb that my biopsy had come back with cancer and I ... *barely nod*. I'm brushing up with my mortality, and nothing is happening. It's almost disappointing.

Instead, I take out a folded piece of yellow paper from

my shirt pocket and a blue-ink pen and prepare to write down notes, as though I'm about to do an interview for a story or make a grocery list. I don't want to miss or forget anything he's about to tell me, so I need to write down *everything*, my memory is so bad. I honestly don't know if I am numb ... or utterly fearless ... or suffering from the shock of just being kicked, you know, *below the belt*.

In fairness, I had read ahead, just in case. Dozens of prostate cancer Web sites and discussion support groups on the Internet told me about an organ and disease I'd known nothing about. I had prepared somewhat for bad news, the what-if scenario that I might have prostate cancer. In the grand scheme of things, there was probably nothing remarkable about this happening to me. The American Cancer Society reports that about 218,000 guys are diagnosed with prostate cancer every year, and about 32,000 die from it, usually because the cancer is discovered in an advanced stage.

From all that I had read, I had about a 95 percent chance of surviving as long as the cancer cells were localized to the prostate, which my urologist believed they were. However, there is always a chance the tiniest molecules of cancer had escaped the prostate undetected, only to find a home elsewhere in the body, likely a bone, and reappearing later.

I figured that the odds were pretty darn good my cancer was localized. Every year for the last eight years, I had taken an annual PSA test, which measures prostate-specific antigen, the protein produced by the prostate. Nothing had shown up until this year. So I had caught it early. The only thing unusual was my relatively young age for prostate cancer. Fifty-five.

Dr. WS tells me one of my 12 biopsy samples came back showing cancer, which I figure was a good ratio. One in 12, okay, how bad could that be? It isn't like I have a huge tumor filling up my prostate. We're talking bits. Microbits.

Just when I start swimming around in the half-full glass, he tells me my Gleason number is 7. Your cancer is on the verge of being *aggressive*, he says. Now at this point, I had only a vague notion of what a Gleason number is ... but the word *aggressive*. That gives me a little jolt.

What I knew about biopsies was that a pathologist examines the biopsy samples and assigns the cancer cells a rating, based on shape and size and how they compare to normal cells. The more ragged the shape of the cancerous cells, the higher the Gleason score and the worst your situation. Having a score of 1-4 is pretty good, 5-7 is the middle ground, 8-10 is the worst case. So I'm thinking my 7 is borderline not-so-great-but-not-horrible. Still, my mind is stuck on his word ... *aggressive*.

Dr. WS then launches into my options, as I start writing it all down, somewhat foggy and disconnected from my scribbles on the paper. He tells me "at my age" I can't afford to wait and see what happens with the cancer. He explains a course of non-treatment called watchful waiting as an option for older guys, usually after age 75, who have the slowest-growing cancer cells. But at 55, I'm relatively young for prostate cancer. So when it occurs, the cancer needs to be dealt with because it can become even more — here it comes again — aggressive. Now he's said it twice!

The cancer needs to come out, he says. You have some treatment options. You could have the surgery … or there's radiation, which is the lesser chance of getting rid of it. (I later learn this is flat-out not true.) But with that comment, he makes it abundantly clear to me that he wants to surgically remove the entire prostate, slice around all my sensitive sexual equipment and peeing apparatus, and pluck it out.

Dr. WS wants the job.

In a somewhat cool and professorial manner, he gives me a primer on the surgical and radiation options, and then he breezes through the risks of each — incontinence, erectile dysfunction stood out — so nothing sounds appealing. While he believes the cancer was localized to the prostate, I would still need a bone scan and CT scan to see if any cancer had escaped the prostate to my bones or my lymph system. But as I'd already read, you never know for sure. Today's most powerful scanners cannot "see" at the cellular level. Even though there's no telling if a spec of microscopic malignancy has split from the prostate, I needed the scans anyway — at best, to see if a larger tumor has taken root elsewhere.

I write all this down furiously, but my scribble looks like a spider web spun on psychedelics. The weight of the moment presses in. *I have cancershit* … he's talking major surgery, my sex life and continence hanging in the balance, not to mention the cancer has to be eliminated, he says. Or else.

In a moment of clarity, I tell Dr. WS I want to talk to a radiation oncologist before making any surgical decision. With the slightest of sighs, he promises to arrange that for me. I want nothing to do with a snap decision. But now I'm also wondering: How long do I have to make this decision before, say, the cancer kills me?

I ask him that, straight out, knowing it's purely roadside rubbernecking on my part. I have no intention of sitting on this news. I have a teenage son, a beautiful wife, a life. Still, I want to know: How long would I have to live if the cancer is allowed to go unchecked? Dr. WS shrugs initially. But I press him and throw out a number: Two years?

Probably, he replies, if you do nothing.

Two years, wow. Could that be? Really? Singer Dan Fogelberg immediately springs to mind. He had just died of prostate cancer. The cancer had migrated to his bones, which a fast-growing and lethal prostate cancer will do. Advanced prostate cancer is a godawful miserable experience, often settling into your lymph system or bones. Extremely painful.

Only two years after doctors discovered it, the music died for Dan.

I could hear my clock ticking.

Before leaving Dr. WS's office that day, I mention a book that another physician had recommended to me, called *90 Days to Prostate Health without drugs or surgery* by Dr. Larry Clapp. Dr. Clapp claimed he had twice cured his own cancer by taking an holistic approach. He used colon cleanses, lifestyle and diet changes, and even removed the mercury from his teeth.

Granted, this intriguing thesis was hardly mainstream, but Dr. WS's reaction is sharply and immediately dismissive, based solely on the title of Dr. Clapp's book. I doubt he read the book. He strongly suggests I read some "real" medical research, and then hands me a book, *The ABC's of Prostate Cancer: The Book That Could Save Your Life* by Joseph Oesterling.

On the cover, it has lot of pictures of famous people who have had prostate cancer. Politicians, a general, entertainers, jocks. So I'm in good company. Deeply appreciative, I say thanks, and leave his office with a heavy textbook to read and weighty decision to make.

Riding down in the elevator, I open the book to its title page and scan down to the date of publication.

1997.

Doc, you gotta be kidding me? I blurt out loud in the elevator, startling a little old man and his wife who had left the urologist's office with me. Even I knew that prostate cancer therapy, especially in the areas of high-dose radiation and robotic surgery, had made giant leaps of progress since then. Why are you giving me a clearly *out-of-date* text to help me make a decision that may affect my life for another 30, 40 years? This is the "real" medical research you want me to read? From 1997... Unbelievable ...

No, this doctor's visit has not gone well at all.

At home, I put on a brave face for my wife, Lorraine, who initially tears up. Then we walk through the good parts of the bad news: We caught it early, and it's the one cancer with the highest cure rate out there. How lucky is that?

As someone who sorts things out in a hyper aerobic state, I head out for a long run and ran into a wall of unfinished projects ... the incomplete novel, getting my son Nick into a good college, no sub-4 New York City marathon, no family white water adventure down the Colorado River, no climb up Kilimanjaro, never jumped out of an airplane, my out-of-date will. Was I leaving enough money behind? Hell, I couldn't even make up my mind where I wanted my ashes scattered? Perhaps the waters straight out from the #4 lifeguard stand on Delray Beach, Florida, where I surfed as a kid and have run by a zillion times? Or the backside of a peak in Colorado, where I skied for 35 years? Which peak? The wise men say 19 out of 20 guys survive localized prostate cancer, but what about the other poor schmuck? Somebody's 1 out of 20. Was that gonna be me?

It was a depressing run.

For the next few days, the weight of the world seems to hang over my treatment decision. I read over and over that no doctor can tell you which treatment will guarantee the best result. No one knows for sure. Both radiation and surgery boast high success rates for the first 10 to 12 years, but after that, it's a tie game; one seems to be just as effective as the other. So you take your chances. Roll the dice.

In truth, the elephant in the room for those with localized prostate cancer isn't survivability. No, it's the risk of collateral damage *as a result of your treatment* — incontinence, impotence, a shrinking penis and, oh, let's not forgot the rectal burn and pooping issues. Quality of life is on the line. It feels like if I screw up this decision, my peeing and sex life may change forever, right to the grave.

At night, I hold my crotch in bed and think, I'm only

fifty-five! I should have decades left of peeing and sex without any special apparatus. No penis pumps, no implants, cracked or not. How did I get to the point of even *thinking* about this stuff? Why are visions of diapers, dribble down my leg, and a bonerless life dancing in my head? Stop!

But I cannot make this suddenly encroaching fear go away.

Three days after my diagnosis, I find myself sitting at a high school baseball game, watching my son, Nick, take the mound in the final inning of a 4-3 game. We're winning. It's up to Nick now, on this beautiful night in early April, to close this thing down. In our quad, three other games had already ended, so all the coaches and dozens of players and parents crowd behind the fence to catch the finish. All eyes on Nick.

All the years of playing baseball, the practices, the travel teams and thousands of hours coaching and playing with Nick — now here he stood, in his full 15-year-old bloom, pitching his brains out on a big game with a big crowd.

A gentle breeze starts blowing in my face and my eyes start to water, as Nick strikes out the first batter, who goes down spinning in the dirt. Then Nick gets the second batter to chase a low outside curve and ground out to second. One more to go ... Nick's on fire.

Suddenly the emotions of the last several days start to wash over me. Nick rears back and fires two fastball strikes and then drops a sick knuckle-curve to punch out the last batter looking. That ends the game. As I watch from the other side of the fence, Nick gets mobbed by his teammates with hugs and high fives … and my eyes start to well up, big ol' fat tears running down my face, until I can barely see him.

> **Blog: April 10, 2008**
>
> About a week after the diagnosis, I finally tell Nick about the prostate cancer. I had waited until making a treatment decision. We sat around the kitchen counter at breakfast. I wasn't sure how Nick would take it. He's fifteen. My intent was to be reassuring, tell him I had a plan. Not to worry.
>
> "Hey, I won't even lose my hair," I tell him, half smiling … waiting. "Any questions?"
>
> He cuts into his waffles, pours a stream of syrup, thinks for a long moment, and finally looks up at me.
>
> "Are there going to be any mood swings?"

The Alternative Medicine Tease

Like most guys, I never gave my prostate a second of
thought until my family doctor pulled on a plastic glove and
delivered my first digital rectal exam at age 47. Drop your
drawers, bend over, a minor discomfort for a few seconds as
he sticks his gloved finger up your rectum about two inches
to the prostate and feels around for any hardness (possible
cancer) and enlargement (BPH), and it's over.

Not a big deal. Get over it.

After that first exam, my doctor told me my prostate
was mildly enlarged, an inevitable result of aging. I didn't
know that, nor did I understand the ramifications of an
enlarging prostate on my entire urinary system.

But in hindsight, I should have recognized the subtle
clues that my plumbing was changing. I recall a car trip with
my son, for instance, when he was eight years old and I was
in my late forties, and we pulled off a country road to take a
leak. Standing side by side, I couldn't believe the huge,
powerful arc of urine he generated, next to my piss-poor
hosing of the weeds. That was a sure sign of an enlarged
prostate at work, squeezing down my urine flow. But I had
no clue.

Why don't men know more about their prostate before
it goes to hell? Does the medical community share any
blame for not educating men early enough? Why are
prostate disorders dismissed as a normal part of aging and
only the symptoms are treated — until things go so horribly
wrong that men need drugs for life or a major medical

intervention?

Why isn't there more focus on preemptive care and prevention? Could men actually reduce their risk and prevent prostate disease and perhaps cancer, with simple changes in diet and lifestyle? This was the question I finally got serious about, though unfortunately, too late in the game to make a real difference.

A couple months *before* my cancer diagnosis, I began visiting an alternative medicine practitioner. Call him Dr. JZ. My symptoms of frequent peeing and burning and leaking and blood in my urine and chronic urinary tract infections were worse than ever, and I was tired of it all. I wanted answers.

Over the years, I had visited Dr. JZ for various maladies that seemed to stump my mainstream physicians. This doctor, also an acupuncturist and herbalist, had pulled off some incredible medical fixes for me, my wife and several friends when no one else could help.

Unlike Dr. W.S., my urologist, Dr. JZ told me on my first visit that he could treat the cause for my prostate issues, not just manage the symptoms. He promised to soothe the storm down under and get at the root of the problem. I found the promise of Dr. JZ's alternative medicine, with its low-tech, non-invasive, benign and natural, herbal-friendly remedies, a very attractive approach.

Although I was excited at the prospects, I was more than a little skeptical, despite his solid track record of fixing the unfixable with his acupuncture needles, strange diagnostic machines and herbal concoctions. Skeptical because I had bought into the general argument that all my prostate problems were due to a "natural part of aging." It had been drummed into my head, and left me with a sense of futility. No regular doctor had any answers for this problem common to so many men, beyond meds for temporary relief. How could Dr. JZ turn back my prostate's clock and actually cure the cause? So while skeptical, I was still willing to try anything, or just about.

First up, he gave me a Biological Terrain Assessment, an exam that measures the "deep health" of the body. A BTA attempts to gain insight into one's overall health by measuring things like body acidity and testing blood, saliva and urine to understand what's going on in the body at the cellular level. In theory, the complete picture of this information gives the practitioner a baseline to build a treatment plan for the underlying cause for illness or disease, rather than treating a list of symptoms. That sounded good to me. No other doctors had ventured into my biochemical/electrical environment to see if they could turn off the spigot of excessive urine and chronic infections.

Dr. JZ also gave me something called a Vega test, which revealed a buildup of toxicity in various organs, including my prostate. He told me this diagnostic machine, with its hand-held electrical probe, could pick up infections, underlying inflammation, toxicity, and other maladies — *but not cancer*. He was upfront about that. For anything to do with cancer, I would need to see my regular doctor for a PSA test.

Based on his readings, Dr. JZ recommended an assortment of teas, organic coffee, antioxidants, high-concentrate beta-sitosterol and nettle root, lycopene, zinc, and vitamin E to cleanse my organs and improve urinary flow. I agreed to acupuncture treatments as well. He also recommended I read Dr. Larry Clapp's *Prostate Health in 90 Days without drugs or surgery*. He seconded Dr. Clapp's advice to consider a colon cleanse and even remove the mercury from my teeth. He was serious.

I bought the book that day.

In *Prostate Health in 90 Days*, Dr. Clapp claims to have actually cured his own prostate cancer not once but twice (yeah, it returned) through an holistic approach — colon cleanses, natural foods, dental care, and de-stressing his life. His argument goes something like this: Over a 70-year lifetime, the average American eats nearly 70 tons of solid food that is over processed, filled with pesticides and hormones, lacking in fiber, and hard to digest. Consequently, many suffer from slow bowel transit time and/or constipation. In clogging up the intestinal pipes, food rots and produces toxic substances and parasites that weaken the body's defenses. Weakened defenses encourage disease. Because of diet-caused clogged colons, toxins leak from the colon into the prostate. This creates an environment for infection and disease and even cancer. So until the toxins and parasites are cleared out of the colon, true healing of the prostate cannot begin.

It's a theory, and I was receptive to it — as a layman desperate for help. The leakage of toxins into the prostate sounded plausible to me, so I waded into the shallow end of his remedies. No, I didn't extract the mercury from my teeth. But I did drink a half-gallon of green tea a day, religiously took twice-a-day doses of complex high-concentrate beta-sitosterol (about 3000 times more potent than saw palmetto), pumpkin seed, white Korean ginseng root, flaxseed oil, and nettle root, antioxidants and vitamins A, E and B6 — and actually began a colon cleanse. What did I have to lose? My prostate was out of control.

After a couple months, my symptoms retreated dramatically. The urgency, starting and stopping, persistent burning and frequency of going to the bathroom 10 to 20 times a day stopped. I started to feel normal again. Ironically, this was also the period when my PSA levels had spiked after an annual checkup, and the possibility of cancer loomed. I went on another round of antibiotics to knock out any infection. While I waited for my next PSA test, I decided to do the colon cleanse as well. I figured, a little house cleaning couldn't hurt, and who knows, maybe Dr. Clapp is on to something, not just promoting a phony cancer cure to sell books. So based on Dr. JZ's recommendation, I bought a specific kit from a distributor in California and started my cleanse in early March 2008.

A couple weeks later, my world flipped with the cancer diagnosis.

Everything changed. No longer was I facing a distressed urinary system. With cancer on the table and the stakes raised, suddenly Dr. Clapp's and Dr. JZ's holistic approach of clean pipes and herbal supplements and acupuncture needles felt like I was trying to slay a monster with a slingshot.

What if Dr. Clapp's cancer treatment regimen, without drugs and surgery or radiation, didn't work? What if I spent months keeping a clean colon and restricting my diet, and even removing the mercury from my teeth (never serious about that one), but the cancer grew and metastasized beyond my prostate? What if I wasted months or a year going down this road, monitoring the cancer by taking frequent PSA tests to see if the level drops? And what if it never goes down? What if, in the meantime, my window of opportunity on life-saving surgery and radiation closes?

The What Ifs. I imagined Dr. Clapp's approach to getting rid of my cancer would be like treading water in a deep, murky ocean at night and waiting to get bumped by that predator shark.

I'd be always on alert for the *really* bad news to arrive. *It's now in your bones, Steve.*

The idea of using low-tech tactics to reverse prostate cancer seemed extremely risky and an agonizingly long-term project, when emotionally and intellectually I wanted to take advantage of catching it early, eradicate it and move on. The "90 Days" way of no drugs and no surgery might have merit — *might* — but at best, I would have turned cancer into a chronic condition that would keep me on edge. Forever I'd be monitoring my PSA to see which way it was moving.

My biggest fear was that by following the "90 Days" approach the cancer would grow beyond the prostate and well beyond the medical choices I had at the time. The book's prescriptions seemed like a great idea *up until* my cancer diagnosis, but once it was in, not so great. Colon cleanses and supplements and dietary modifications and dental work come off as a weak attack on a lethal enemy.

So when circumstances got serious for me, I turned away from Dr. Clapp and Dr. JZ. I returned to my mainstream doctors to help me confront cancer.

Nevertheless, I came away from the whole flirtation with holistic healing and BTAs and Vega tests and acupuncture believing that alternative medicine might do a better job at addressing the problems of the prostate *before* cancer appears.

The experience left me thinking if I'd more conscientiously nurtured a healthier prostate years earlier, perhaps the symptoms wouldn't have manifested at all — or, at least, they might have been more manageable. Perhaps the cancer itself could have been prevented.

At my time of peak desperation for answers, I didn't question the veracity of Dr. Clapp's claims that he cured his own cancer — twice! — through holistic regimens and lifestyle changes. Maybe I should have, maybe the claims were outrageous. Certainly my mainstream doctors, like Dr. WS, thought so.

But for me, whether Dr. Clapp is on the trail of a radical cure-all or not, it just didn't matter when the cancer appeared. The consequences of gambling on an alternative, unscientific protocol — and failing — seemed way too high.

I just couldn't take that risk.

And as I was learning in all-things-to-do with prostate cancer, it's all about settling in with the risks you're most comfortable taking.

The Therapy Menu: Pick Your Least Fear

The first and most important thing I learned as a newbie prostate cancer host is that no single therapy has proven superior over any other. That blew me away. The realization unnerves you in the first few days after a diagnosis when you're looking for your doctors to advise you on the best road to take to, ostensibly, save your life.

The fact that physicians are uncertain about which treatment is best — and that the patients will have to exercise their own best judgment in deciding on a treatment — is one of the aftershocks of a prostate cancer diagnosis for many men. It sure was for me. I couldn't help but wonder, why isn't there more consensus on one *best* treatment?

The easy answer may be that every prostate cancer patient brings in different variables: age, stage of cancer, lifestyle choices, risk tolerance. The scientific research is inconclusive, plus the technology for new treatments changes at lightening speed. All the data isn't in place for mainstream physicians to speak about *what's best* with absolute certainty.

In the end, the patient has to consider the many variables and weigh them against a smorgasbord of treatment options. Every treatment comes with its own mixed bag of unpleasant side effects, primarily urinary, bowel and sex-related. The patient has to imagine the life *after* treatment, which often makes the decision process confusing, frightening, intimidating.

But no one can tell you what's *best*. For dockworkers and lawyers and bakers and English-major writers like me without medical degrees, this is a revelation. *It's your call.*

So every guy needs to do his own homework. All men diagnosed with prostate cancer have to weigh the pros and cons of various therapies, none of which look great. So be deliberate — and, most important, think ahead.

As Dr. Ronald Wheeler, a noted urologist, prostate disease specialist and medical director of the Diagnostic Center for Disease in Sarasota, Florida, wrote in his book *Men at Risk, a Rush to Judgment*, "You cannot accept the consequences of your decision until you fully understand the lifestyle you have to accept when the choice is made."

That, if nothing else, is for certain.

Your menu of therapy choices. Pick your least fear:

Watchful Waiting

This is a euphemism for doing nothing, except monitoring your situation. Men over 75 years of age often make good candidates for watchful waiting, because their cancer is generally slow to grow and rather harmless. Less so for younger guys, say in their 40s and 50s and 60s. Their cancer *tends* to be more aggressive and *probably* requires some form of aggressive treatment.

One theory goes that younger men's bodies produce higher concentrations of dihydrotestosterone, a byproduct of testosterone, which fuels the growth of prostate cancer. The older you get, the less dihydrotestosterone you have, resulting in a slow-growing cancer and a diminished need for aggressive treatments like surgery or radiation.

That, however, may oversimplify the issue.

New research has found 28 strains of prostate cancer, about 15 percent of which are considered fast growing — and age may have nothing to do with their rate of growth. For that group, expecially those with at least ten years of otherwise healthy living ahead of them, watchful waiting may be a risky option.

By choosing a path of watchful waiting, you would not undergo any active treatment. No medications, no radiation, no surgery. Instead, your doctor monitors your prostate cancer with regular PSA tests and digital rectal examinations. These tests keep an eye out for changes that signal your prostate cancer is growing more quickly, which might call for aggressive therapy.

For older men, it's not uncommon that the cancer neither spreads nor causes any symptomatic problems, hence watchful waiting makes good sense. For younger guys, watchful waiting can also be a rational option as long as they remain vigilant, know the facts, and accept the risk of a tumor spreading and becoming incurable.

Radical Prostatectomy Surgery

Most urologists, being surgeons, would prefer to do what they're trained to do — surgically remove your prostate rather than turn you over to a radiation oncologist. The rationale for surgery is fairly straightforward: Cut out the entire prostate, cancer and all, before it can spread.

Unfortunately, no one can guarantee you that the cancer

hasn't already escaped the prostate. Even with the most powerful high-tech scanning equipment, no one can "see" whether microscopic bits of cancer have taken up residence beyond the prostate. So don't believe any advisor, even one with medical shingles, who says surgery will "get rid of it," as I was told. It might not.

A radical prostatectomy, long considered the "gold standard" in the surgical treatment of prostate cancer, is a major operation and carries a high risk of side effects. Surgeons must cut around bundles of delicate nerves and blood vessels involved in urination and ejaculation. Depending on the size and location of the cancer, nerve-sparring surgical procedures may be used to preserve much of those functions. But again, no guarantee.

Nerve-sparring surgery certainly sounds a whole lot better than the unthinkable (and medieval) alternative. But even with the nerve-sparing approach, those precious nerves webbed around the prostate can be damaged or destroyed. Although some men recover completely, impotence is a potential complication after any surgery, even with recent improvements in prostate removal. Urinary continence is another possible complication. After surgery, most men need a urinary catheter for a week or two, and some must wear absorbent pads for a few weeks. Most men are fully continent within a year.

Typically, men diagnosed with prostate cancer under age 60 are steered toward surgery because it's believed to offer the best chance for long-term survival. But this standard advice might not be best for everyone — or even true anymore. New high-dose, targeted radiotherapy and proton therapy have become increasingly effective and might do a better job at minimizing risky side effects.

Da Vinci Robotic Surgery

A higher-tech variation of a radical prostatectomy is called da Vinci robotic prostatectomy surgery, in which a machine actually performs the cutting while a surgeon operates it remotely. It's become extremely popular, now accounting for more than 86 percent of all prostatectomies.[1]

With a human surgeon at the controls, the da Vinci system filters out hand tremors, enhances precision, offers 3D imaging and seems to eliminate some of the fatigue associated with conventional laparoscopy. In theory, by using finer tools to make smaller incisions, the robot can do better than a surgeon in removing the prostate and minimizing the collateral damage.

A high level of skill is generally required, so pick a surgeon with lots of experience with da Vinci, because experience directly relates to successful outcomes. Otherwise, you become, as one of my doctors warned me, "a data point on some doctor's learning curve." With your sex life and normal peeing functions in the balance, you don't want to be anyone's guinea pig.

Radiation

If your doctor is a radiation oncologist, expect a recommendation for radiotherapy, or radiation treatments, instead of surgery. Radiologists have their own bias toward their area of expertise, just as the urologist-surgeon does. They both believe in their years of training and the science behind each treatment, but pressed, neither specialist knows if one treatment offers a better chance of survival than the other.

Radiation therapy uses high-energy X-rays to eliminate cancer cells and shrink the prostate. Radiation doesn't kill the cells immediately, but instead destroys them when they attempt to divide in two. Given that it takes a while to kill the cancer, treatments generally take place over extended periods of time, usually eight or nine weeks.

You can choose from many flavors of radiation therapy.

The old standard radiotherapy approach is called **external beam radiation**, in which the patient lies on a table and radiation is beamed externally over the abdomen. The technician delivers the radiation over a large area in case the cancer is more widespread than the prostate itself. In this shotgun approach, the radiation can spill over from the prostate into neighboring organs, tissue and internal plumbing, which can cause a litany of common side effects: incontinence, diarrhea, fatigue, irritate bowel syndrome, skin irritation, nausea. Of course, even with a more generalized approach, you can't be positive the radiation will kill all the cancer. Even if one cell got away, it can grow again and spread and you'll likely have to try a different "salvage" therapy other than radiation. Too much radiation can actually *cause* cancer, so generally, you get one shot at radiation as a cure-all.

Internal radiation, or **brachytherapy**, involves tiny radioactive seeds (about the size of a grain of rice) implanted into the prostate. The idea is to keep the radiation *inside* the prostate rather than passing it through the body and possibly harming sensitive organs and tissues. The seeds give off small amounts of radiation for weeks or even months. They are left in place after they stop emitting radiation.

The side effects of brachytherapy differ from external beam radiation. The seed implant method can deliver a higher dose of radiation to your urethra (the tube passing through the prostate carrying urine from the bladder), so negative urinary symptoms after treatment tend to be more severe and long lasting. Most men tend to suffer more frequent, slower and painful urination. Some men require medications or even intermittent self-catheterization to urinate. On the positive side, rectal symptoms may be less frequent and less severe with brachytherapy compared to external beam radiation.

High-dose radiation therapy, the latest and more targeted approach, comes in different forms. The most popular is intensity-modulated radiation therapy (IMRT) and image-guided radiation therapy (IGRT). IMRT and IGRT techniques use a special CT scan and computer to precisely aim the radiation in the prostate. These high-dose therapies promise to leave vital organs and healthy tissue near the tumor unaffected. Unlike conventional radiation, these techniques manipulate the radiation to the shape of the prostate, protecting the bladder and rectum from radiation scattering into those areas. The intended result? Significantly fewer side effects.

Proton beam therapy, a form of targeted external beam radiation, is also gaining in popularity, as providers build more and more quarter-billion-dollar facilities the size of a couple football fields. The attraction for patients is that protons, unlike X-rays, pass through healthy tissues with little damage and destroy only tumor cells in their path. In theory, proton therapy not only reduces side effects, but it saves more lives.

Critics say proton therapy is exorbitantly costly, and, to recover the cost of investing in the technology, providers could be over-treating elderly men who'd be better served by watchful waiting. That criticism, by the way, applies to expensive high-dose radiation therapies as well.

Other therapies

Cryotherapy freezes the prostate in order to kill off clusters of cancer cells. Side effects are considered rather mild, although the big risk is impairing sexual function, so I suppose it depends on your definition of "mild." The freezing of the prostate might destroy the nerve bundles responsible for erections. Cryotherapy may be a good option for high-risk patients or those who haven't benefited from previous radiation therapies.

However, there is a new super-cold cryo treatment that is garnering some serious attention. Called **focal cryoablation**, it allows doctors to freeze cancer cells at negative 40 degrees using 3D biopsies to target the treatment directly to the tumor. The big promise is that it kills the cancer without invasive surgery and without the usual side effects, and can be delivered in a single, outpatient treatment. Radiation and other therapies can take weeks or even months.

High Frequency Ultrasound, or HIFU, is the opposite of cryotherapy's cold therapy; it uses high-frequency sound waves to heat the cancer cells and destroy them. It was first used by the Chinese and is now available in Europe, Mexico and Canada, and in clinical trials in the U.S. for patients who've experienced radiation failure. HIFU is a treatment that because it's based on sound waves, it doesn't have many side effects like other treatments.

Hormone therapy involves using drugs or surgery to remove the testicles. That stops the body from producing male sex hormones (androgens), which are believed to stimulate the growth of prostate cancer cells. Hormone therapy works by either preventing the body from making these androgens, or by blocking their effects. In either case, the hormone level drops, slowing the growth of the prostate cancer. Hormone therapy is often recommended in combination with radiation and sometimes surgery.

Photodynamic therapy is an experimental treatment to keep an eye on, or at least ask your doctor about. Here, doctors inject patients with a medication that adheres to blood vessels supplying prostate tumors. Next, they laser off cells, resulting in a blood supply loss to the cancer cells. This treatment kills cancer cells in a single, outpatient treatment.

Best advice on this menu of treatment options? Talk to your physician about these and other choices. Prostate cancer technology is advancing in leaps and bounds, even vaccines are under development. Do lots of homework and don't jump at the first option presented, even by a trusted physician.

Remember, even when prostate cancer is caught early and is most curable, a successful treatment — or one without side effects — is not guaranteed. Every man should understand all his options and choose the best one suited for him, based on age, cancer stage, and risk tolerance for potential lifestyle side effects.

> ### Blog: June 27, 2008
> Making the decision on how to treat prostate cancer was easily the most stressful period of the whole cancer experience. The diagnosis got my attention. But digging into doctors' heads, doing my own research, and aligning heart-head-and-gut on making the right decision … therein lies the grinding stress and anxiety. By comparison, the nine weeks of therapy was a sleep walk.

Betting All My Marbles on a Cure

So what to do about my prostate cancer: Get blasted with two million times the amount of radiation as a dental X-ray? Or allow a robot to cut open my crotch and carve out the malignant gland?

Over those two completely unappealing options, I spent every night for a week after my diagnosis losing sleep. The Internet, especially the prostate cancer discussion boards and online support groups, is an excellent place to freak yourself out beyond all reason and common sense.

Oh sure, I read lots of success stories. But most of them were Stephen King nightmares. Browse through all the botched surgeries and sloppily radiated lives, listen to guys talk easily about catheters and penile implants and diapers, and you can't help but reach for another Ambien.

Before consulting with the radiation oncologist, I called my family physician and several doctor-friends, and asked these trusted medical experts what they thought about the radiation versus surgery debate.

What would you do if you were me?

Two were internists, one a neurosurgeon, the other a urologist. All of them echoed the same advice: Based on the facts that I'm relatively young for prostate cancer and otherwise healthy, my Gleason score a borderline-to-aggressive 7, cancer grade T1c, and the cancer caught early and likely localized to the prostate, they all said surgery.

It was standard guidance for a guy my age. The advising urologist told me if he were in my position, he'd want to know it was gone, so he'd cut it out and "be done with it," he said. (This, as I learned later, was somewhat misguided, since there's no guarantee, even with localized prostate cancer.)

Adding in the vote of my urologist/surgeon Dr. WS, all those in favor of surgery 5, radiation 0. Nada one.

Next stop: the radiation oncologist, Dr. BG. I admit, I did not like the idea of a bloody surgery (even if it was a nerve-sparring operation), a catheter hanging out my penis for weeks after, and then living in suspense for a year wondering if I would be impotent for life.

Nor was the da Vinci robotic surgical approach — of making clean, small, precise incisions to open me up before scalloping out my prostate — an attractive way to go. Surgery in and around my urinary and sexual apparatus just spooked me. The post-surgical catheter, plus diapers for months to absorb the leaking, made it all seem worse.

So the day I walked into Dr. BG's office a week after the diagnosis, I was hoping to hear about a less invasive, bloodless, catheterless alternative.

We talked for a full hour — the doctor, Lorraine and me — in a small patient room in the cancer center. Just as my urologist had done, Dr. BG gave me a guided tour of the treatment landscape, carefully emphasizing the benefits of radiotherapy over surgery, but not because the odds would be better for survival. They weren't. He admitted the cure rates were about equal: five-year survival rates nearing 100 percent for both radiation or surgery for early-detected, localized prostate cancer.

I had done enough reading to think I might be a strong candidate for brachytherapy, in which radioactive "seeds" are implanted in my prostate and emit bubbles of radioactivity to zap the cancer. This seemed like a very cool option to me. No surgery. No daily radiation treatments. Once implanted with seeds, the radiation takes place without me doing anything. I radiate on the run and at work. I radiate and kill cancer cells in my sleep. I just need to stay away from pregnant women for six weeks or so. Not a problem.

However, Dr. BG didn't think that brachytherapy would be the right therapy for me because my 7 Gleason score was too high. Instead, he thought I'd be a better candidate for the latest in targeted, high-dose radiation — imaged-guided radiation therapy, or IGRT. He said it would give me the same certainty for survival as if I had my prostate surgically removed: 10 years of being cancer free.

Beyond that? "Intuitively," he told me, "we believe that IGRT will be as good if not better than surgery over the long term and without the side effects."

Dr. BG explained that over the last ten years radiotherapy for prostate cancer had gone on an Apollo Moon mission of sorts, in terms of technological breakthroughs.

With IGRT in particular, the usual spillage of radiation outside the prostate — compared to earlier external beam and brachytherapy delivery systems — has been minimized from several centimeters down to one or two millimeters. That's like narrowing the Grand Canyon to a crack in the sidewalk. The promised result of this precision is that IGRT saves the bladder, protects the urethra, and largely avoids sensitive sexual apparatus from getting singed and scarred by radiation.

In the spring of 2008 when I consulted with Dr. BG, IGRT was very new — the cutting edge. First introduced in 2003, it uses an automated imaging system to obtain high-resolution three-dimensional images to pinpoint tumor sites and adjust the patient's position on the table when necessary. That too was a huge and important breakthrough.

Before IGRT, radiation oncologists had to deal with daily variations in patient positioning, including internal organ movement. Bladder filling, for instance, could alter the center of the prostate, and the location of the cancer from day to day. With any changes like that, the risk of side effects increases.

By contrast, IGRT enables doctors to locate the tumor before each dose is administered by locking on to four gold "markers" that are implanted into the prostate before treatment. Even if the prostate moves — say, from gas bubbles or urine in the bladder — IGRT uses the gold markers to adjust daily to the new position. The dosage can even be regulated within the radiation beam to avoid highly sensitive areas like the urethra that carries urine from the bladder.

All of this sounded pretty good to me — at least compared to the blood and catheters and hospital stay of surgery.

Once I was convinced the cancer was not likely to kill me anytime soon as long as I did *something*, my decision on treatment focused on one thing: what therapy offered the least risk of collateral damage in the peeing and sexual activity departments? Once you can say that 10-year survivability is a virtual certainty, a tie game, whether you go with surgery or radiation, then the only thing left to talk about are the side effects of the therapy; primarily, incontinence and impotence.

Here again, surgery came out a big loser, at least in my mind. All the doctors except the radiologist had counseled me to seriously consider surgery — which I did. But it seemed crazy. The risks atrociously high — around 15 to 25 percent higher chance for some combination of incontinence and impotency, compared to high-dose radiation. At 55 years old, these were horribly unappealing odds.

"It's a no-brainer," my brother, Kurt, said flatly, after talking through the options and risks with him.

And, in the end, I agreed.

(The Prostate Cancer Foundation and other groups constantly update statistics on the short- and long-term treatment risks on urination and sexual function. The good news is that newer technology and better procedures are lowering the risks of incontinence and erectile dysfunction, whether you choose surgery or radiation.)

Before leaving Dr. BG's office that day, I had one last question about high-dose radiation. Seeing that my biopsy had revealed a prostate sick with prostatitis and BPH too, would the radiation wipe them out as well, and all of their annoying and inconvenient symptoms? He was careful with his answer — I sensed he didn't want to over promise an outcome. But he seemed *more than hopeful* that the radiation would clear up the other two diseases while killing the cancer.

A three-fer-one? I know he basically said "maybe" but that's not really what I heard: No, I left that day thinking IGRT would fix all my bewildering plumbing sins — all in one fell swoop of sizzling, cell-frying, infection-blasting mega-radiation.

I'm in.

Walking out of Dr. BG's office, after a week of dreadful hand-wringing and anxiety and fear bubbling up about what to do next — I felt an enormous weight lifting from my shoulders. My gut and heart and head all locked up in sync, the gears grinding into alignment, on one game plan.

Yep, I knew what I wanted to do: I pick IGRT. So super radiate me. I'm ready to bet all my marbles on it.

Fact was, no one had proven to me beyond a doubt that surgery offered better long-term survivability than the latest advances in radiotherapy. All my doctors seemed to agree that the chances for survivability were about equal through 10 to 12 years. After that, no one could say.

They seemed to be recommending surgery because it had been the 'gold standard' treatment while high-dose radiation was the new and unproven kid on the block. I think some doctors felt trying something so new was a gamble. The data just wasn't in yet on this new radiation. But with an "aggressive" cancer at my door, I couldn't afford to wait years for the data to arrive. I had to go with my gut.

Interestingly though, no one seemed to dispute that high-dose radiation would offer me less risk, in terms of minimizing collateral damage to my plumbing equipment and sex-related apparatus. And that is what I had become most concerned with: My lifestyle *after* treatment.

At the time, I scoured all the research I could find, and began to look at collateral damage as a percentage game. In other words, 55 percent risk of erectile dysfunction after two years with surgery, compared to 30 percent with radiation … 15 percent less risk of incontinence with IGRT … almost no risk of rectal burn with surgery, 2 percent with radiation. Those were the numbers I was dealing with. So you make all of those comparisons, and then do what makes the most sense.

You pick your least fear.

Shortly after the consultation with Dr. BG, I visited my urologist, Dr. WS, and told him I wanted to go forward with radiation, not surgery. I couldn't tell if he was disappointed to lose my business, I suspected he was. I didn't bother to tell him that if I had decided on surgery, it would have been the robot not human hands, certainly not *his* hands, doing the cutting. He may've been a great doctor, but I didn't completely trust him ever since he gave me that old prostate primer book from 1997.

Dr. WS asked me about my thought process, why at my age I would want to go *against* conventional wisdom and not have surgery. I told him, simply, I thought both would kill the cancer. My concern was collateral damage. I worried about surgery killing my sex life.

Surprisingly, he just nodded, and didn't bother to put up a last defense for his specialty. Shortly after, I thanked him again for the *ABCs of Prostate Cancer* book he'd lent me, lied about how it'd been a big help, and left. His reaction to my decision, and my gut sense about it, made me feel like I'd made the right choice. But to be perfectly honest, at this point, I was desperate not to be wrong.

Blog entry: April 4, 2008

Hours after the diagnosis, Lorraine tells me, weepy eyed, "You know, I always thought maybe you'd fall off a mountain skiing... but nothing like this," referring to my termination by prostate cancer. Now really, how cute is that? And what am I to think of it? Every year, despite her concerns for my demise at high altitude, she's always very encouraging that I go on those annual ski trips with the guys...

Blog entry on exercise and reducing prostate cancer: April 21, 2011

Run, walk, bike, sweat a little — guys treated for prostate cancer can reduce the risk of prostate cancer reoccurring by over 60% with three hours a week of vigorous exercise compared to men who got less than one hour per week of vigorous exercise. These findings came from the Health Professionals Follow-Up Study of 2705 men observed every two years over 18 years. "Vigorous" simply means "a very brisk pace" — in other words, work up a sweat for 30 minutes a day, six days a week. For anyone who has gone through surgery or radiation and all that anxiety about how things are gonna turn out, a little exercise every day is a small price to pay (and a cheap insurance policy). Why the positive outcomes from all that exercise? The study's authors suggest physical activity might influence cancer survival by modulating insulin activity and inflammation and/or by altering the immune system's behavior. More research is required. Source: **The Washington Post**, "Exercise may extend life after prostate cancer diagnosis," January 1. 2011.

Manning Up for the Gold Marker
Implants (and Earlier Biopsy)

The first step in obliterating the cancer through IGRT is to implant four permanent 24-carat gold pellets — about the size of a grain of rice — into the prostate.

The pellets are key to creating the perfect kill zone, in that they allow a computer to lock onto an exact position of the prostate, day after day, before deadly radiation is delivered in concentrated doses. (Why 24 carat? The better the gold, the less interaction with human tissue, I was told. And no, the pellets won't set off metal detectors in airports.)

The procedure to insert the pellets is similar to a biopsy. After a local anesthetic, an ultrasound probe is placed up the rectum. The probe allows hallow needles to poke through the rectum wall and into the prostate. There, a computer visualizes the whole scene and allows the doctor (or technician) to place each pellet in the right spot. A breeze, right?

Well, in my world, anesthetic or not, anything going up my rectum is going the wrong way. Still, I have cancer, I'm trying to get rid of it. It's time to man up, even if this feels anything but manly.

In truth, neither the marker insertion nor the biopsy is all that traumatic with a good nerve block. I know, because I had both — a good one and a bad one.

In the biopsy, the mystery and awkwardness of it all may have been the worst part. Slipping into a hospital robe, I hop on board a table, lying pretty much naked on my side, my rear-end pushed out — the ready position. Talk about feeling vulnerable. The room light is low so Randy, the medical technician, can easily view an ultrasound of the prostate area on an overhead screen.

First the local anesthetic. He probes my anus with an eight-inch-long needle until he finds just the right spot along the rectum wall and squeezes — a sharply painful fire exploding up my rear. Don't want to be a weenie here, but that shot hurt like hell. I got two of those, just to make sure; the second not as painful.

Next, Randy inserts the ultrasound probe in my anus. Into that, he inserts a device that punctures through the wall of the rectum and into my prostate, and begins snipping. Twelve tiny pieces of prostate come out, one at a time, each piece of tissue bitten away with the sharp sound of a metal SNAP! Each time, I keep waiting for a painful jolt to follow. But it doesn't happen. The local nerve block does its job.

Of course, because the biopsy was performed before my diagnosis, I had not entertained a treatment decision or what that might entail. So that day, I climbed off the table and got dressed again, thinking I'd had my one and only cigar probe and knitting needle stuck up my butt. Thank God for that…

But only weeks later, after the biopsy came back positive and I'd decided on IGRT, I had the gold marker insertion done.

Back on the table, ready position.

This time I somewhat know what to expect, so the mystery had faded. Same low-lit room, same Randy the med tech (joined by my radiologist this time), same nakedly vulnerable position on the table, same eight-inch needle for a local anesthetic, same kind of ultrasound probe maneuvered into position up my rear. The only thing significantly different between the biopsy and the marker insertion is the numbing effect of the nerve block.

The shot, uncomfortable as ever, just doesn't take — not completely.

The first two implants are okay, a little bloody as it turned out, but not bad. But as the third of four markers go in, I almost fly off the table. A live nerve! Don't move, don't move, Randy tells me, with some urgency. But how could I stay perfectly still when a hot-pointy delivery device, thick enough to carry a rice-sized pellet (the gold marker), pierces non-anesthetized nerves up my rectum? They asked if I wanted another shot of the nerve block. And I'm thinking, Do I want that needle sticking my rectum wall again? That's gonna hurt like a bitch too, so what's the point, there's only one insertion left.

No thanks, I tell them, just get it over with.

So as they prepare to insert the fourth marker, Randy quite seriously offers this bit of instruction: Rather than recoil with the pain, he said quite seriously, try to sink your butt into it and hold the position, hold as long as you can, so the pellet can be placed in just the right spot and we don't have to go back in.

Ready? Oh, I'm ready. As ready as anyone can be for a

rectal electrocution.

As the fourth marker went in the same way as the third, I do my job and hold my position, while the doctor fiddles inside my prostate with the perfect placement of the last gold pellet. Oddly, the pain feels almost good, *almost*, because it's the kind of hurt that precedes long-lasting relief. It's the point-2 in a 26.2-mile marathon; you know it's almost over, you see the finish line.

So I do the only thing I can do. I closed my eyes. Stop fighting it. And relax, pushing down into the pain.

> ▶ Blog: April 21, 2008
>
> Today I watched an exciting Boston marathon, and when the cameras turned to Lance Armstrong, all I could think about was running in next year's Boston and getting an entry through Armstrong's Livestrong Foundation by raising money for prostate cancer research. So I went on the website, looking for ways in. I'm thinking, get through the cancer... and start training for Boston's 113th next April. That or NY in the fall.
>
> With a Boston/NY run in my head and radiation starting in four days, today I'm getting an ultrasound on the mysterious blackness behind my knee — what my orthopod and Dr. BG thought might be a Baker's Cyst, possibly caused by a slight meniscus tear. I probably need some kind of outpatient surgery on the tear.
>
> The ultrasound, he told me, is just preventative, to rule out any vascular problem. So I'm heading there now... and thinking about another marathon as a bookend to this cancer.

Time Out for a DVT:
Cancer's Hidden Danger

I barely had time to wrap my brain around having prostate cancer — and the perilous risks of treatment and painful gold-marker implants — when things took a sharp turn,
from bad to shoot me.

Not long after the cancer diagnosis, I visited an orthopedic surgeon for a strange, bruised, squishy protrusion
behind my left knee. The doctor thought it might be a
meniscus tear, but had to rule out anything more serious, so
he sent me to a radiologiest for a scan of my leg. An ultrasound scan revealed a monster in the midst — an eight-
inch-long blood clot in a major vein in my upper calf. In
med speak, a deep vein thrombosis, or DVT.

The radiologist who found the massive clot showed
more alarm than Dr. WS did when he delivered the cancer
news — and for good reason: Unattended prostate cancer
might kill you in maybe two to eight years. The clot ... *in
the next 60 seconds.*

The radiologist told me to rush — don't wait, go now,
RIGHT NOW! — to my family doctor who would stabilize
the clot, a jelly-like mass floating in the blood soup of a
deep vein. He'd stabilize it before a little chunk could break
off and move to my lungs where it could be fatal. Pulmonary
embolism.

The clot is big, the radiologist said. How big? Well,
think eight inches of twined yarn from your knee down into
the upper calf. Do you feel any pain in your chest or

shortness of breath or have you coughed up any blood? he asked. He's looking at me a little too wide-eyed for my state of mind, which is controlled panic. No, I told him. Good good, now go … GO!

Talk about a lousy bedside manner. The guy made me feel like I was sitting on a time bomb about to explode ... *any second now* ... maybe even while driving to my family doctor's office! This is insane! I had yet to ask the why-me question when it came to the cancer; I didn't want to be a self-indulgent wimp who couldn't handle bad news, even if it was malignant. But this potentially deadly DVT that I'd barely heard of before and could tear loose any moment and wind its way up the blood-river vein to my lung and that would be it. C'mon, man. In football, this is piling on. I thought it was a tiny meniscus tear.

Okay, I mention the DVT in the middle of this cancer story, not because this is my lousy luck, but because blood clots are potentially part of every cancer story, particularly prostate cancer. Some two million Americans a year are diagnosed with DVTs, and up to 30,000 die from them. Yet the incidence of developing a DVT increases dramatically for cancer patients.

In fact, prostate cancer patients have double the risk of suffering blood clots that can lead to a DVT and pulmonary embolism. In one study,[2] scientists looked at more than 76,000 Swedish prostate cancer patients who received curative treatment, or hormone therapy, or were being monitored without treatment. All were found to be a higher risk of blood clotting than men in the general population. This risk is especially high for younger men — less than 65 years of age, the boomer population — and men with advanced prostate cancer.

This 10-year study shouldn't have been a surprise to anyone in the medical field. Earlier research has linked cancer with the risk of blood clotting. Past studies have shown a person with cancer is four times more likely to develop a clot than a healthy person, although the reasons are not clear.

Strangely (in hindsight), none of my doctors made mention of potential clotting, nor did they connect the dots — the blackening swollenness behind my knee, the diagnosis of prostate cancer, the higher risk for DVTs. No warnings, no conversation about clotting risks, nothing. Yet I was showing the weird fat dark spot to all the doctors who were consulting me on the cancer. To his credit, my radiologist Dr. BG told me I needed to see an orthopedic physician to get it checked out. But even he lacked any sense of urgency, and we didn't talk about the DVT at all.

The damn thing hurt too, like a severely strained calf muscle, something I might have to deal with following a marathon. Still, the soreness and black puffiness behind my knee all happened at the same time as the cancer diagnosis and the preoccupying treatment decision. At that time, attending to a painful calf was down my list of priorities.

> **Blog: April 24**
> A friendly warning to anyone suspected of prostate cancer — or any kind of cancer for that matter:
> *A blood clot may try to get you first.*

After the DVT was discovered, my family doctor immediately gave me a shot of the drug heparin, which stabilized the clot within an hour. The risk of a piece breaking off to my lung was over.

Then, instead of being hospitalized, I opted to give myself daily Heparin injections in my stomach for five days to affix the clot to the vein wall. I also began a six-month regimen on the blood thinner coumadin (also called warfarin, an anticoagulant) that kept the leg from developing another clot.

Crisis averted. Now what? How long before the eight-inch snake goes away?

My doctor's answer of a year or two, or never, was not what I wanted to hear, so I contacted a top researcher on DVTs at the National Institute of Health. Dr. Richard Chang told me that about half of all DVT patients have positive clinical results, meaning no pain and no swelling, after 3 to 6 months of treatment. But he warned me that the coumadin only thins the blood, it won't dissolve the clot. A natural enzyme in the blood, called tissue plasminogen activator

> **Blog: April 28**
> Note on DVTs: About 85 percent of air travel thrombosis victims are athletes — mostly endurance athletes, like marathoners. People with slower blood flow are at greater risk of clotting. Also athletes are more likely to have bruises and sore muscles that can trigger clotting. Not surprisingly, clots often go misdiagnosed. Like mine, the clot often feels like a muscle cramp or a tight knot. So aggravating the injury and increasing the risk of permanent disability or death is higher among athletes than other groups.

(tPA for short) flows over the surface of the clot to break it down naturally. Over time. Lots of time. As long as the clot is only partially occluding the vein — as opposed to a full occlusion or blockage — blood will most likely dissolve the clot. In the meantime, Dr. Chang told me, be patient. Wear compression socks to facilitate blood flow in my calves.

Ironically, the day after discovering the clot, it sunk in about the good timing of the DVT event. Obviously, no clot-chunk had broken off to my lung. But if the DVT had been found *before* the bloody markers insertion, Dr. BG would have delayed the radiation treatment, maybe six months. That would've been stressful. I wanted to get it over with, kill the cancer. But he wouldn't have taken the risk of me bleeding out internally on the blood thinners.

My first morning injecting a needle full of heparin in my stomach, it occurred to me how lucky I was to find the DVT when we did.

Yeah, real lucky. *Now squeeze…*

> **Blog: April 23**
> Trying to wrap my head around blood clots and cancer, blood thinners and radiation treatments, kidney stones (found in a CT scan)… against all this, Nick saved his first District game as a sophomore, 1-2-3, to preserve a 6-3 win. Awesome performance! Before he pitched, I got a little emotional, the weight of the week I suppose. I asked him for a lift, and he delivered. Two saves on the night — one for the team, the other for his dad.

Radiation Day Eve: Meeting Carol

A couple of twenty-something female medical technicians in seafoam scrubs — one a perky brunette, the other a pony-tailed blond — shave my pubic hair at the edges and tattoo the clearing with a "plus" sign, and then they burn permanent blue dots on each of my hips. I'm pretty much naked. They're ridiculously cute.

I lie under a hulking IGRT machine, the cutting-edge of high-dose radiation therapy that I hope will kill off my prostate cancer and, if I'm truly lucky, my other plumbing miseries. I'm betting on it, in any case. Inexplicably, the women call the machine — my high-tech savior and, with some irony, my potential emasculator — Carol.

This is Radiation Day Eve. They are prepping me.

Carol is a stunning piece of technology in her own right, this IGRT or Image-Guided Radiation Therapy machine. Imagine a sand crab the size of a Hummer with three giant claws that hover and whirl and click around my body and will radiate my microbits of cancer to death over nine weeks, five days a week.

Today I lie on a table in the mouth of the crab, my hospital robe scrunched up to my chest, no underwear, a loin cloth, white socks. The two female techs have fit me to a custom molded half-body cast to keep me perfectly immobile. I will need to lie absolutely still so my pelvis can be correctly CT-scanned and beamed with up to 7750 centrigray of radiation for about 90 seconds each session. (By comparison, an X-ray at the dentist's office is about .14

centigray, about 50,000 times less than my daily dose.)

To line up Carol with my pelvis, red rays of light will crisscross my three micro-tattoos, creating a perfect killing zone to whack the cancer.

As the techs pick delicately around my loin cloth, I'm suddenly feeling scared. And why not. I have prostate cancer my doctors have called aggressive. I'm only 55. A lot of normal living is at stake here. So, of course, I'm scared — of the big technology overhead, of whether it's gonna do its job and not wreck the plumbing and sexual apparatus. But mostly, I'm scared of these female techs fingering around the edges of my groin and how this is gonna go. To be perfectly frank, I'm not thinking cancer right now, I'm not concerned about my mortality one bit ...

No, I'm on high alert that my penis might, you know, suddenly move — dart, twitch, roll over — under their gaze. How embarrassing would that be, any slight, you know, *woodening*. I'm a happily married guy, but everything is SO sensitive right now and some things are just out of my control. I close my eyes and focus as hard as I can. I'm trying to will it: *Penis*, don't move, don't go rogue on me, not now. *Behave.*

Eyes shut and concentrating, I hear the two techs talking softly to one another. I don't know what they're saying, exactly, so I take a peek, and oh no, now they're taking measurements around my groin, oh please, with a ruler ... gorgeous young women staring at my pubic area measuring things. C'mon.

It's cold in here too. Their hands are cold. Which brings this thought: *What if they're now staring at a bump of flesh, a wee shrunken nothing.* Just as I think about which is more mortifying, these strange cute girls seeing my penis twitch or seeing it shrunken up to tortoise head, the blond covers me with my robe flap and cheerfully tells me to relax a few minutes. Steve, you're all set …

Yeah. Relax. All set.

And just like that, they turn and bounce out of the room to leave me alone to my thoughts. I'm lying half inside the claw, in the middle of this large windowless radiation room, my home for the next nine weeks, the lights turned down low. I stare at walls with hanging cameras and the indecipherability of the IGRT machine, and I'm blown away by it all, how I got here, and how helpless I feel lying here, soon to receive massive amounts of life-saving radiation on an organ I knew zero about only a month ago. Sure, I've read and learned a lot since the diagnosis, but just like every other aging male, the prostate is mostly a mystery. Its encroaching miseries, and the cancer itself, caught me completely by surprise.

I close my eyes again, and let my mind go. A mid-fifties boomer, a whole post-midlife of normal continence and sexual functioning rides on the outcome here; it rides on the tattoos and measurements these young, gorgeous medical technicians just took.

Flat on my back, I'm suffering a form of buyer's remorse. In the choice between surgery and radiation therapy, I obviously elected to go with the latter, and against considerable expert medical advice that I didn't agree with. But honestly, what the hell did I know? I made this decision in a matter of weeks. Should I have just cut it out and be done with it, as all my doctors, except my radiologist, recommended. Will radiation spill over and fry my rectum and bladder? Is my life of boners about to end? Should I have done nothing instead? Am I one of millions of guys being overtreated? Maybe another pathologist should've read that biopsy? Is it too late to crawl off this table and go home to reconsider my options?

But I don't.

I just lie there, thinking what a huge leap of faith this is, because *no one knows* what the best treatment is for prostate cancer. While my odds of surviving are extremely high because it was caught early, no doctor knows which therapy promises a better cure rate, or which treatment will produce the least amount of collateral damage. It's a percentage game.

As far as I was concerned in that moment, nobody knew anything and this was all a huge gamble.

It felt like I was laying down the biggest bet of my life. Despite all the medical advice I'd sought out and all the careful research I'd done, the gut checks and family counsel — the best I could do is cross my fingers and hope like hell that I'd made the right treatment choice and I'd been tattooed in the right spots.

Lying there, marinating in fear and doubt and alone under the high-tech tonnage of Carol, I hoped, I prayed, I sucked it up. It's all I could do.

Beam On: Getting Radiated

I began radiation treatments on a Monday, in late April 2008. Monday through Friday at 4 p.m. for 45 weekdays, I got super radiated. I got weekends off to rest and let my body bounce back from any accruing fatigue. I received a concentrated dose of 7750 centigrays of radiation each day over the first few weeks, decreasing to 5000 centigrays a day for the last five weeks. I will only receive a radiation treatment once in my life for this cancer. Quirky fact for those of us without medical degrees: A second go-round with this much radiation could actually cause cancer.

Every day I walk into the cancer center, I take a locker, strip and don one of those backless hospital robes. I sit and watch Dr. Phil on a television and chat with the other guys. All of us wear blue or green robes. Every fifteen minutes a voice comes over the intercom, announces a name, and the next guy proceeds to the radiation room. I'm the second to the last guy of the day. The other guys are all older than me by a generation, at least. Most are in for prostate cancer, others for throat cancer. Unlike me who works all day, most of the men I meet are in for a late-day radiation treatment so it doesn't conflict with their morning tee times.

When my turn comes, I clutch the back of my hospital robe and walk into a hallway and through another door and into the huge radiation room. I'm supposed to be completely naked, except for the robe. But after a couple of treatments, I wear my socks and boxers. It's freaking cold in there. To hell with the rules.

In the center of the radiation room is Carol, the giant IGRT machine. The same two young and cute female techs who prepped me bring me my custom-fitted, half-body cast to lie in, and they fuss around me as I get centered on a table under the machine. I slip my boxers down to my knees, and we go through this ballet where they allow me to place a cloth over my loins. Red lights from the walls lineup across my three tattoos. The girls lean in and stare, making sure everything is just so. Sometimes they take measurements, of what I don't know. For the first days, I felt, well, modest. Then I got use to it, and I started flopping around and hanging out without a care. Whatever. Let's get on with it.

The girls finally leave the room. Within a minute or two, the three giant claws of the IGRT machine start whirling, clicking and roaming around my body. The IGRT then locks on to the gold markers inside my prostate, scanning images and sending them to a computer in the next room, then moving again to another position and re-aligning, grinding loudly before a buzzing sound starts up and an electronic display box on the wall flashes ... *BEAM ON* ... in bright red lights.

> **Blog: May 17, 2008**
> Trust me on this one, if you smoke STOP TODAY!
> My radiation buddy Larry, 78, is a lifer smoker
> undergoing radiation twice daily plus chemo for his
> throat cancer. His face is burnt red and blistered, and
> his throat is filled with open sores from the radiation,
> so he can't eat. He lives on a feeding tube. He swears
> a lot. "This is fuckinhell," he tells me.

When I see the red lights, the big claw is radiating me!

I hold my breath every time. I'm afraid of moving my prostate with a gulp of air. The girls assure me I can breath, but why take a chance — these are my margins of error we're talking about, a silly millimeter of radiation slop that could burn my bladder or rectum. They tell me to stop worrying, to breathe.

But I hold my breath for 10 to 30 seconds for each radiation blast. I get eight blasts per session, totaling maybe a minute and a half. That's it. Over that period, the radio-therapy exposes my cancerous cells to controlled doses of radiation, damaging their DNA. Because prostate cancer grows slowly, many weeks of therapy are necessary to continually damage the DNA in the bad cells. And therein lies the beauty and wonder of radiotherapy: Normal cells also get zapped, but they're able to repair the damage — cancerous cells cannot. So my doctor tells me. Yes, all cells take a beating, but the bad guys die off and the good guys rise from the ashes. Amazing.

All of this, from robe on to robe off, takes about a half hour a day, if that.

> **Blog: May 28, 2008**
> On my weekly Wednesday consult with my doctor, Dr. BG, I ask the Harvard-educated radiation oncologist how the cancer is doing after almost five weeks of concentrated, focused, high-dose killer radiation. "By now," he says to me, "it's wondering, *what the hell is going on here*." Now that's a professional analysis ...

What's it feel like? Does radiation hurt? Burn? Tickle? I'm asked that a lot. The answer is no. The actual delivery of mega doses of radiation feels no different than sitting in a dentist's chair getting an X-ray. Which is to say, not at all.

The cumulative effect of daily radiation, however, can creep up on you. Every day a nurse weighs me, in case I start dropping pounds. I didn't, some men do. I rarely had complaints, and took some pride in that. My energy stayed pretty strong and steady, likely because, as a runner, I entered therapy fitter than most, my radiologist told me. Fitter than most? I'd hope so. The youngest patient after me was 20 years my senior.

Like running long distances, I monitored what's going on in my body. Fatigue is the biggest complaint of prolonged radiation exposure and I did get draggy a few times by the

---

> ### Blog: May 20, 2008
> The guy who gets radiated before me, Mr. Gregory, is a 70-year-old African-American guy who has lost two brothers and his dad to prostate cancer, and a third brother to lung cancer. He didn't want to have the surgery because "if I can't screw anymore, what's the point."
>
> He has a girlfriend. Once when she came over to his house, dirty dishes were piled up in the sink — very uncharacteristic of him. When she asked how's he doing with the radiation, he pointed to the sink and said, What's it look like?
>
> "I use to be compulsive about things like dishes — now I don't give a shit. The cancer's helped me relax," he told me.

end of the week. But I didn't dwell on it. If I get fatigued running, I slow down. If I got tired from the radiation, I took a 20-minute catnap. I might do that once a day, and I was good to go.

Once I had four to five days of diarrhea, another common side effect, but that cleared up on its own. My only steady complaint was a persistent urinary burn by week three, so I stopped running, which seemed to irritate things, and began swimming laps four times a week in a pool. Happily, some of my old symptoms from the chronic prostatitis, like the frequency to urinate, the burning and persistently annoying drip that spotted my khakis, seemed to clear up.

Once a week after treatment, I sat down with Dr. BG, who always told me the radiation zapping my cancer was "spot on." He told me that he studied the CT scans and printouts of my treatments every night, monitoring every nuance of the therapy. The only thing he didn't do was the daily set up and pull the lever to radiate me. He was nowhere to be found for the actual deed.

> **Blog: May 24, 2008**
> Not bitching and moaning here, but: Week four of
> radiation sucks. My stools broke up and diarrhea
> ensued. I pee fire. It feels like I'm ejaculating razor
> blades. I'm told the full prostate radiation ends
> next week — and the radiation will focus on smaller
> areas in the prostate, leaving the urethra to cool down.
> One of the guys in the Waiting Room tells me his burn
> subsided after the fifth week.

You cannot understate the level of my anxiety when I first realized medical technicians — the two female techs who fixed me up every day, and three others on computers — were assigned that task, and not the guy with the shingles from Harvard. Nobody mentioned that. But by the time you figure it out, there is no turning back.

> ### Blog: May 31, 2008
>
> Larry, with the tongue cancer from a lifetime of smoking, walked into The Waiting Room after treatment this week and declared that the doctors told him that after double-sessions of radiation for eight weeks, his cancer was gone. "My God, this shit really works!" he said, which made us all laugh. Waiting Room humor.
>
> Several days later, Larry finished up his treatments, and while I was thrilled to see him cured, it was oddly bittersweet knowing Larry wouldn't be hanging out in the Waiting Room anymore. Watching the Closing Bell on CNBC. Swearing the occasional blue streak. He may've been in his late 70s, me in my mid-50s, but the difference in age hardly mattered when you're fighting the same battle.
>
> "The doctor says in a month I can eat a pastrami sandwich. You know what it means for a Jew to be separated from the deli? It hurts right here," he says, pointing to his heart, just above his feeding tube.

> Blog: June 28, 2008
>
> In many ways, I found the experience of cancer had less to do with the disease itself and more to do with the love you experience from others. I think that's why you'll hear so many cancer survivors say that their cancer was a gift. I use to think, **What are you talking about? Cancer a gift? Hell, it's trying to kill you...** But I kinda get it now, all that unsolicited love and kindness flowing your way. It overwhelms, and it leaves you grateful.

The Aftermath: On 'Roids, Rectal Burn, ED, Dry Orgasms and Skydiving

Almost two years after my cancer treatment, I find myself flying in an open gutted-out Cessna at 13,500 feet along the edge of the Florida Everglades. Just ahead of me, the high winds whip at my son, Nick, now poised at the open bay door. It's a stunning blue summer day in South Florida, puffy white clouds floating in flotillas far below us. Nick's about to jump.

It's his first skydive, I go after him. My first jump too. An old friend, Roy, will follow behind me. We're all fastened in tandem to an instructor on our backs. We're celebrating Nick's 18th birthday and my PSA returning to normal with a two-mile freefall at 120 miles an hour, followed by a 3,000-foot float under an open parachute to a drop-zone back on earth.

Nick has his game-face on, I've seen it a million times, while pitching on a baseball mound, all unflappably cool and focused. Only now instead of a baseball uniform, he's wearing a goofy blue jumpsuit and pointy black helmet with huge Adam Ant goggles. I can see his eyes though, narrowing as if to make the vastness outside the plane smaller.

As he moves forward into place, Nick's knees slide over the wide black line at the edge of the open bay door. He's positioned almost half outside the plane, buoyed by his tandem partner. Ready to go. Hanging over the abyss. His *Moment of Holy Shit* has arrived.

I can't take my eyes off him. This is more compelling than my own MOHS just seconds away. When he was four, this boy threw a fit and cried refusing to ride Dumbo at Disney World. And now this! He pushes out his tongue, in some high-flyin' Jordanesque move, staring down into the vast middle distance outside the Cessna, and with nowhere else to go, he grins just enough, and ... *dives*.

My turn next.

I slide on my knees to the open door and look out, trying to find Nick. He's long gone. This is the first time I've done anything to push the envelop, to crash the barriers of routine maintenance, since I finished 45 days of radiation therapy for prostate cancer two years ago — which is disappointing. Not the radiation, I have no regrets there. But doing something edgy ... adrenal filled. I had planned to run a marathon, my 14th, as a way to reclaim my body and my old adrenaline-junkie mid-50s self, within months after the treatment, but those plans fell apart.

The problem had more to do with lower back problems from a physically active life that caught up with me, rather than with the cancer therapy, which went pretty well. Six consecutive PSA tests dropped and settled just around 1 ng/ml, which included a predictable (but still anxiety-ridden) PSA bounce to 1.9 ng/ml before settling back down to my nadir, or low point, near 1. The low PSA was an excellent sign and prognosis of things to come. But once you have cancer, you keep tabs on it for life, on the chance a malignant cell may have escaped the prostate and started to metastasize somewhere else. Chances are the low PSA means something else will kill me (like this jump), and what a relief that is.

Lucky me, in facing the prostate triple-whammy of BPH, prostatitis and cancer, my therapy may have actually delivered a *three-fer*. Meaning "three for one" — all three conditions wiped out in one fell swoop of high-dose radiation. Two years later, so far, so good. There's no more frequency all day and night. No burning while peeing, no dribbling, no leaking. No more urinary track infections. Even the plague of jogger's hematuria — blood in my urine — has cleared up, though admittedly the running mileage isn't near what it used to be. Amazingly, my urologist gave me a digital exam six months after the radiation and described my once enlarged and inflammation-riddled prostate as "smooth, supple and small."

I'll take it.

My original pathology report showed my prostate had

been filled to the brim with prostatitis and BPH, along with specs of cancer. The infection and inflammation may still be hiding out in the recesses of my prostate, since I still have one, but the old miserable and inconvenient symptoms seem to be gone. Like I said, a three-fer.

The jury is still out on my sex life, or at least how high functioning it will be without drugs. Months after the radiation therapy, I learned I have to wait out five years to see if I am among the 50 percentile group that has no lingering effect or only mild erectile dysfunction. For the other half, the ED is more severe. In making my treatment decision, somehow that little tidbit escaped my due diligence, and certainly no doctor pointed out the risk was that high. So I'm passing it on here.

I still wake some mornings with drug-free boners, just like the old days. I've become a hoarder of free samples of the very expensive Viagra, Cialis and Levitra for mild ED, all of which effectively engorge a stimulated penis with blood for sustainable erections. Before taking the samples, erections weren't the same. They became flaccid in a hurry, and this was freaking me out. So the extra help is welcome, and I don't sweat the fact I need to take a pill. The radiation, as with the surgical options, often and likely destroys too many sensitive nerve bundles related to sexual function. I say, accept it going in to treatment and be grateful the Boomer credo of "better living through chemistry" has yet another wonderful application for our senior, post-prostate cancer years: sustainable hard-ons.

Radiation's collateral damage also extends to a new orgasm, the so-called dry orgasm, a misnomer in my case. It isn't really *dry*. It's a semi-dry orgasm, which only means the milky seminal fluid once made by the prostate no longer exists. I squirt a clear-as-spring-water substance, which is pure semen. I'm surprised how little semen is actually produced, maybe a tenth or less of your old volume of ejaculated fluid. Good news, though. The orgasms feel pretty much the same, just less juice.

After extensive radiation treatment, some men experience the phenomena of shrinkage as well. That's when the boys don't hang as long as they once did, another factoid the urologist and radiation oncologist will likely omit from pre-treatment discussions. No matter. Honestly, I don't believe it has any functional relevance; you look like you're exiting a cold pool. It's — ahem — a small price to pay.

The worst of my treatment aftershocks, as it were, was the radiation burn on my rectum and the DVT in my lower calf.

First, my ass on fire: Because my cancer grew on the outer edge of the prostate bordering the rectum, radiation spilled over and burned my rectum wall — despite the promise of the precise, targeted delivery of radiation to the cancer. Oh well. A millimeter of radiation slop from my prostate to rectum wall was just enough to burn and scar misery up my rear end.

I knew this was a risk up front. Dr. BG, my radiation oncologist, warned me about rectal burn, but added the chances were minimal, something like 1 in 50 patients. When cancer is knocking at the door, you take your chances.

During my post-treatment summer, I suffered serious

rectal burn and raging hemorrhoids. My family doctor told me I might have to have surgery to repair the damage. But he advised me to wait it out for several months to see if the problem would heal by itself.

Over the next four months, I lived on prescription suppositories, Metamucil, stool softeners and handfuls of ibuprofen to try and reduce the inflammation. My ass was a scorched mess, as if the blowtorch just couldn't be removed. I avoided business meetings. At home at my computer, I sat on a big cushy donut that looked like a toilet seat. It barely helped.

Insanely, I actually tried to train for a marathon through all of this. Doomed to fail, I ran anyway. I really wanted to run in the New York City Marathon to cap off my cancer experience. I thought I'd contact Lance Armstrong's Livestrong Foundation and try to raise money for cancer research. Only days after my diagnosis, the race and the cause seemed like a great idea. It gave me a lofty goal. I also had a guaranteed entry from the previous year's lottery. Mostly, I loved the notion of reclaiming my body from the grip of cancer by completing a marathon. During treatments, I swam nearly every day and worked out with weights to stay strong, ward off fatigue from the radiation, and get ready for my marathon training when the therapy ended.

I'd completed 13 marathons so I knew what it took to get ready for 26.2 miles. To make what would be my third NY start at the foot of the Verranzano Bridge in November, I would need to train for a good 18 weeks following my nine weeks of radiation. With treatment to end in June, the timing couldn't be more perfect, it seemed. So days after my diagnosis, I paid my $165 entrance fee to New York. I was in. The only thing left was to get through the treatment and then train my ass off.

Ha. What I hadn't planned on, of course, was post-treatment rectal fire for the entire summer, plus my cranky back, and, oh yeah, the DVT in my calf. As I began putting together a few 20- and 25-mile weeks between hemorrhoid flare-ups, my leg with the eight-inch-long DVT swelled up like a balloon. The clot occluded normal circulation through the lower leg, which fattened with volumes of blood during and after my runs. I wore compression socks to help facil-itate the circulation through the leg, but that didn't solve the problem. The clot was just too big. While running, my leg couldn't keep up with the increased blood flow, and it would expand easily one-third larger than the other leg.

Hot ass, fat calf ... I kept running. But in my post-treatment pursuit of reclaiming my body from cancer, my physical challenges wouldn't go away. First, a CT scan back in March discovered a couple kidney stones, so I had a lithotripsy to shatter them with sound waves; then an unrelated pinched nerve in my lower back knocked me off training for enough weeks that I finally trashed my marathon plans. Too much downtime.

My marathon comeback plans and fundraising for the Livestrong Foundation, noble goals as they were, died a slow death through the summer. Sometime in September, I canceled my entry to run New York. Just not my year.

The hemorrhoids and rectum miseries finally settled down after four months, and disappeared for good after six months. The DVT is an ongoing problem, but it's slowly wearing down from passing blood, as will a rock under a century of rains. As the researcher at the National Institute of Health told me, the clot will dissolve if you give it enough time.

One year after therapy ended, I developed overactive bladder syndrome (OBS), likely the result of radiation touching the bladder as well, and it took a long while to manifest symptoms. How terribly annoying. At first, I thought it was the reappearance of BPH or dreaded prostatitis because of the frequent trips to the bathroom again during flare-ups. But a new urologist thought it might be radiation burn. He told me OBS from radiation burn becomes chronic in one-third of patients, often in their second year after therapy. The other two-thirds of sufferers grows out of it. Luckily, that appears be me. After many 10-day to month-long bouts with OBS, it too has thankfully gone away.

As a writer, I wish I had some profound and stirring insight from my cancer experience that I could put down on paper and it would read as if I'd returned from the Light with shareable wisdom for all. But I don't. Or I wasn't paying close enough attention.

But here's the thing: Before the cancer, the thing I prized most in my life was the time I spent with my family, Lorraine, and my son, Nick, coaching him and his friends at youth baseball, and when he moved on to high school, watching him play and pitch without ever missing a game.

After the diagnosis, I realized I'd been doing it right, for the most part, focused on the important stuff: my family and friends. My big revelation on having cancer was how incredibly generous and thoughtful people were toward me with their love and concern. So many people sent me prayers, positive thoughts, good vibes.

I was overwhelmed by it all.

Many of the people praying for me were complete strangers too. An old college buddy of mine had become a Baptist minister, and he had his entire congregation sending up prayers for me on Sundays. "They're talking to God on your behalf," he'd tell me. A five-year-old boy named Joseph, the son of a longtime business client, put me in his nightly bedside prayers for months on end — yet he'd never met me. Email prayer cards flowed in, with people constantly reminding me they held me in their thoughts and prayers.

Lorraine and Nick, they were my oxygen as I went into that deep dive that is cancer. I breathed their kindness, love and concern every day as I watched the sacrifices they made to help me deal with everything. They were awesome.

If anything jumped out and grabbed me by the throat, it was that cancer reminded me to be more grateful for all things in my life, material and otherwise. Mainly otherwise. My cancer gift heightened a sense of gratitude.

Still, I started fantasizing about an adventure as my two-year anniversary after therapy approached. Thankfully, many of the side effects of the radiation seemed to have worn off. All that newfound gratitude aside, I had an itch that had gone unscratched with the trashing of my marathon plans. Some alternative ideas: climbing Mount Rainier came to mind, so did bicycling across the country, rafting down the Colorado River, powder skiing in the Caribous, buying a big, loud Harley and heading to Alaska.

With Nick turning 18 and heading off to start college, what I really wanted was to do was something with my son. Something to satisfy the adventure bug and live a moment together we wouldn't forget. Short on time and cash to prepare for scaling a mountain or the motorcycle trip to Alaska, why not jump out of an airplane?

Two and a half miles up in the sky, I'm staring down at a patchwork of farms and glades, as the Cessna rumbles along at 90 miles an hour. My fists hold firm the straps running up my chest, and I shake my head that I'm ready to go, the adrenaline pumping. Time to fly. Is this what I was searching for? I try again to spot Nick somewhere below, but he's disappeared into the tapestry.

I duck my head underneath a low bar in the open door, and inside a flash, I'm out the plane, plunging headlong in freefall down the elevator shaft, my arms outstretched in flight, chest-to-ground position, wind screaming in my ears, *total* sensory overload. My brain just can't quite grasp what's happening around me, until, after maybe eight seconds we reach terminal velocity of 120 miles an hour, and a cushion of air suddenly supports us enough for my tandem partner to spin us left and then spin right and then swing off this way and that, surfing the high winds.

At around 3,000 feet, eye level to the clouds, I pull the

ripcord and we pop open for a seven-minute float back to earth. "Welcome to my office," my instructor says in my ear. From all hell breaking loose, it's now serenely quiet. He manipulates the chute as we corkscrew down to an emerald green field with a gravel bulls-eye in the middle of it. I can see Lorraine, looking up and waving. Even my Mom is down there waving.

I wave back, still dropping.

We come down steeper than I thought we would. I raise my legs, but just as we're about to touch ground, my instructor tells me to extend them again — I do, and we almost make a smooth landing before tumbling in the long grass, the chute blowing over us. Not a soft, clean landing by any stretch, but with a guy strapped to my back, it could have been ugly.

Getting to my feet, I unhook from the instructor and chute, and see Nick making his way across the field with a big smile, and I start walking toward him, both of us like a couple kids at the endorphin carnival. Beaming, we find each other in the middle of the open green field and slap a high-five, as Lorraine and Roy, who landed before me, now make their way toward us, all grins. Everybody is all grins. As thrilling as the initial leap out the plane was, as satisfying as a marathon finish might have been, I couldn't help but think how perfect this was: Standing in that field, sharing a big moment filled with slap-happy joy and hugs and a huge adrenal release, with the ones I love.

For that — and for not peeing in my pants out of fear or anything to do with my prostate — I'm genuinely grateful.

Part 2
PROSTATE 101

The Mystery Gland

Okay, before moving on to the basics of prostate disease, the risks, the connection to diet and inflammation in the body, and what you might consider eating to nurture a healthier prostate, first a word about the mystery gland itself.

The prostate plays a crucial role in the male reproductive system. Found at the base of the bladder (about two inches past the anus), the prostate gland secretes seminal fluid that combines with sperm during ejaculation. This fluid acts as both a lubricant to help prevent infection in the urethra and as a booster to energize the sperm.

The prostate starts out as an almond-sized gland, until puberty, when it doubles in size. This growth is fueled by male hormones called androgens. Testosterone, the main androgen, is made in the testicles. The prostate stays at a normal adult size as long as male hormones are present. After around age 45, the prostate starts growing again, and for some men, it grows for the rest of their lives. That growth is made up of benign — non-cancerous — tissue, which can grow inward, outward or both. That condition is known as benign prostate hyperplasia, or BPH.

In a plainly horrible design, the prostate surrounds the upper part of the urethra, the tube that carries urine and semen out of the penis. So anytime the prostate enlarges inward, or grows from infection or inflammation, it squeezes or constrains the urethra. Hence, the annoying symptoms of a sick prostate: frequent urination, weakening stream, inconvenient dribbling, burning, urinary tract infections and assorted issues that make urination more difficult.

Bundles of sensitive nerves that help cause an erection of the penis envelop the prostate like spider webs. Treatments that remove or damage those nerves can cause, to varying degrees, impotence or erectile dysfunction. This is why when men are told they have prostate cancer, they need to seriously look at the potential impact of surgery, radiation, or other therapies on those nerve bundles.

> Journal: January 15, 2009
> The inevitably sick prostates of boomer guys represent a lucrative market, from drugs for BPH and prostatitis to cancer treatments such as high-dose radiation, da Vinci and proton therapies. These high-tech remedies generate big bucks for hospitals and physicians. Providers, of course, take on big risks, as today's expensive treatments can become obsolete in a blink. Is recapturing their huge investments NOW contributing to overtreatment (especially in older guys)... instead of recommending more watching and waiting? Makes you wonder. My guess is, until a better screen can discern lethal from nonlethal prostate cancer, overtreatment will persist and the prostate will grow as a huge profit center for providers...

Blog entry: May 2011
Boomers in the crosshairs —the stats

- Prostate cancer is the most common non-skin cancer in America.
- One in six American men will be diagnosed with prostate cancer.
- In 2010, more than 218,000 American men were diagnosed with PC, with more than 32,000 American men dying from it. That's one death every 16.4 minutes.
- A man is 35% more likely to develop PC than a woman is to develop breast cancer
- Approximately 2 million American men currently have prostate cancer.
- A non-smoking man is more likely to develop prostate cancer than he is to develop colon, bladder, melanoma, lymphoma and kidney cancer combined.

Risk Factors, Symptoms and Screening

- African American men are 56% more likely to be diagnosed with prostate cancer than Caucasian men and are nearly 2.5 times as likely to die from the disease.
- The only well-established risk factors for prostate cancer are age, ethnicity and family history of the disease; however, high dietary fat intake may also be a significant risk factor.
- The chance of being diagnosed with prostate cancer increases rapidly after age 50. More than 65% of all prostate cancers are diagnosed in men over age 65.
- Early prostate cancer usually has no symptoms and is most commonly detected through PC screening tests such as the PSA blood test and digital rectal exam.

Survival Rates

- Prostate cancer can be eliminated from the body by surgery or radiation if diagnosed at an early stage. However, every year, 70,000 men require additional treatment due to a recurrence of prostate cancer.
- Because approximately 90% of all prostate cancers are detected in the local and regional stages, the cure rate for prostate cancer is very high—nearly 100% of men diagnosed at this stage will be disease-free after five years.

Projections

- The number of new cases and deaths of prostate cancer is expected to increase dramatically over the next decade as baby boomer men age into the target zone for prostate cancer. If there is no change in prevention or treatment strategies by 2015, there will be approximately 3 million men battling prostate cancer. If there are no better treatments or a cure for prostate cancer by 2015, 45,000 men will die from the disease each year.

Source: Prostate Cancer Foundation

BPH and Prostatitis: Your Warning Shots

Old guy joke: Men spend the first half of their lives making money, the second half making water. Ha. Prostate humor.

Like clockwork, most guys past age 50 eventually find themselves, like me, trudging off to the bathroom all night long or heading to the urinal with two minutes left in the fourth quarter. They face an array of inconvenient and annoying prostate issues — mostly noticeably excessive peeing.

Call it the guy's curse. All American men, if they live long enough, will experience some kind of prostate disease and prostate cancer before they die. And that may mean dealing with all the issues that involve a faltering, neglected prostate — from frequency (gotta go all the time) to urgency (*feels* like you gotta go all the time) to hesitancy (takes forever to get going) and even painful ejaculation (self explanatory).

The most critical issues always surround a guy's ability to have normal sex and normal urination — the kind and quality you've always taken for granted most all your life.

The worst case scenario is, of course, prostate cancer. Only lung cancer causes more cancer deaths among American men. With nearly 218,000 new cases diagnosed in the United States in 2010, about 32,000 men died from the disease, according to the American Cancer Society.[3]

Most of the big cancer research organizations report that prostate cancer will be diagnosed in 16 percent of men, and that its prevalence increases in older men — and increases *significantly*. From the National Cancer Institute:[4] "By age 50, one-third of American men have microscopic signs of prostate cancer, and by age 75, half to three-quarters of men's prostates will have cancerous changes."

Importantly, they go on to say, "Most of these cancers either remain latent, producing no signs or symptoms, or they are so slow growing, or indolent, that they never become a serious threat to health."

Johns Hopkins Research has reported similar findings from autopsy studies, revealing microscopic evidence of prostate cancer is found in 15 to 30 percent of men over the age of 50 and in 60 to 70 percent of men who reach the age of 80.[5]

Many researchers report even higher incidence with advancing age. Among them, the University of Virginia Health Science Center in 2009 reported it believes prostate cancer incidence is possibly as high as 80 percent by age 80.[6]

The Prostate Cancer Research Foundation says that based on autopsy studies all men who live long enough will develop prostate cancer — 100 percent after age 100. You get the picture: *The prostate, as it ages, is a breeding ground for cancer*, at least in the U.S. and Europe and other Western countries.

Before moving on to *why*, let's take a look at what can go wrong with your prostate first.

Odds are the first signs your plumbing is going haywire is because of **benign prostate hyperplasia**. BPH refers to a slowly progressive enlargement of the prostate. It can make urination painful or difficult and send men shuffling off to the bathroom many times during the day and night. Although BPH affects the prostate, physicians often refer to resulting symptoms as "lower urinary tract symptoms" or LUTS. These symptoms reflect changes on urinary flow that extend from inside the prostate, causing pressure on the bladder. Hence, the LUTS diagnosis.

While not believed to be life threatening, new research identifies BPH as a disease of systematic inflammation and, therefore, many speculate it's a potential precursor to prostate cancer. This remains highly controversial, however. For years, chronic inflammation has been documented as an increased risk factor for BPH, but only recently has it been viewed as a major factor in prostate disease progression.[7] Most mainstream doctors hesitate to link BPH with cancer, even as forensic scientists almost always find BPH and prostatitis alongside prostate cancer in autopsies.

Prostatitis is often extremely difficult to treat, largely because the disease appears in several forms. Some prostatitis patients experience acute episodes, with sudden and continuous pain that lasts for days. More common is chronic prostatitis, which may last for weeks, only to disappear and flare up again. Prostatitis is further differentiated by bacterial and nonbacterial causes. Nearly 95 percent of patients are thought to develop prostatitis from nonbacterial causes.

Prostatitis has been famously called the "waste basket of clinical ignorance" by Stanford University urologist Dr. Thomas Stamley because of the difficulty in diagnosing and effectively treating the disease. Also, because the symptoms of prostatitis are so similar to BPH, many doctors don't distinguish between the two diseases and treat them similarly.

Typically, most patients receive a prescription for an antibiotic to manage their disease. Rounds of antibiotics are often used to quell the inflammation and reverse what can be incredibly painful symptoms, particularly during acute episodes. Patients are grateful when it works, but the relief is usually temporary. For sufferers like me, the only thing that seems permanent is the cycle of antibiotics, relief, and more antibiotics when the disease flares, which spawns infections in the urinary tract or bladder. It's a treadmill of misery.

Although prostatitis and BPH can be painful, annoying, inconvenient and embarrassing, they are the lesser of the three evils.

Prostate cancer itself is the most common non-skin cancer found in American men. Prostate cancer results from mutations in the DNA of cells that cause those cells to grow and divide rapidly. The underlying cause for those mutations is still unknown, although chronic inflammation has become a serious contender. Other key risk factors include genetics, aging and a high-fat, sugary diet ... which causes inflammation in the body.

While the number of men diagnosed with prostate cancer has increased in recent years, prostate cancer death rates began to decline and level off several years ago. Many experts attribute the decline to the routine use of the PSA test and because men have become more aware of prostate cancer and are acting sooner.

It is a virtual certainty that men will first have to deal with the discomfort and frustration of either BPH and prostatitis, or both, before prostate cancer appears on the scene. Most primary care physicians still discount any linkage between the three. My doctors told me there simply was not enough "hard science" to connect BPH and prostatitis as causes for prostate cancer. A growing body of research, however, shows the three prostate diseases may be linked as diseases of chronic inflammation.

Both BPH and prostatitis should be taken as warning signals of danger ahead, of serious changes underway in the prostate, rather than unlinked diseases. In fact, these two "benign" conditions may be the harbingers for cancer, the canaries in the proverbial coalmine.

The Inflammation-Cancer Connection

You can go back to an early 19th century researcher named Rudolf Vinchow, head of the institute of pathology at the University of Berlin, who first popularized the idea that inflammation was a predisposing factor to generating tumors. This idea fell out of fashion for decades. However, over the last 10 years or so, the inflammation-cancer connection has undergone a renaissance of sorts.

Johns Hopkins Research, for example, has advanced the theory that inflammation may be a "smoking gun" for prostate cancer development.[8] According to pathologist Angelo De Marzo and others on the Johns Hopkins team, the idea is that chronic inflammation leads to tissue injury and ultimately to oxidative damage. This, in turn, leads to mutations in DNA, and mutations lead to cancer. [9]

As a result, De Marzo and the Johns Hopkins Research team have called prostatic inflammation "a primordial potential breeding ground for cancer." What these researchers are finding is that in the thick of cancerous and precancerous cells are hotspots of inflammation, where cells are growing out of control.

This is not unlike what scientists have found in other cancers. Long-term inflammation is known to cause damage to cells and to DNA and is associated with many kind of tumors. Chronic stomach inflammation causes stomach cancer, chronic hepatitis causes cancer of the liver, and reflux esophagitis can progress to cancer of the esophagus.

The latter example happened to my dad. He spent most

of his life sucking Tums for persistent heartburn, a chronic irritation of the esophagus. That irritation eventually turned into a more advanced inflammatory condition, Bartlett's Syndrome, which evolved into esophageal cancer, which killed him.

Another leading researcher, urologist Dr. J. Curtis Nickel of Queens University, Canada, has also written that it is the chronic, persistent nature of inflammation that damages cells, especially cellular DNA, and causes genetic mutations that lead to uncontrolled cell division that characterizes cancer. Adding more fuel to the fire, urologist Timothy Moon, of the University of Wisconsin, has reported that 100 percent of the surgical and biopsied prostate cancer specimens he has examined show the presence of prostatitis.[10] Again, this indicates that inflammation underlies the prevalence of prostate cancer.

This notion of an inflammation-prostate cancer link has been supported over the years by plenty of indirect evidence as well. In a four-year study of 8,231 men age 50-75, for example, the drug dutasteride (Avodart), used to reduce the size of an enlarged prostate, has been shown to reduce the risk of prostate cancer by 23 percent in men with an increased risk for the disease.[11] In another more recent study at Washington University School of Medicine in St. Louis, men who take dutasteride have up to a 40 percent chance of not being diagnosed with prostate cancer compared to those men who don't take it.

Taking an aspirin a day has many health benefits, and reducing prostate cancer may be one of them. New research from the University of Texas and presented at the annual meeting of the American Society of Radiation Oncology in 2009 shows men who use aspirin or other blood thinners after treatment for prostate cancer have a substantially lower risk of dying or seeing the cancer spread to another organ. The study followed 5300 men with prostate cancer. In those taking blood-thinners such as aspirin, only 4 percent died from recurrence of cancer after 10 years, compared to 10 percent who did not take the medication — reducing the risk of dying from cancer by more than half.

Johns Hopkins Research cites population-based studies that found lower prostate cancer incidence among men taking inflammation-reducing medications or following diets less likely to promote inflammation. Additionally, the organization Cancerhelp UK includes aspirin and anti-inflammatory drugs as factors that may lower risk for prostate cancer.[12]

These studies that indicate anti-inflammatory drugs can reduce the risk for prostate cancer are noteworthy. Why? Because using them may help avoid the high costs and the devastating side effects of unnecessary surgeries and radiation treatments, or it may help men prevent recurrence of cancer.

Like many men, I suffered through the symptoms of chronic prostatitis (inflammation) and BPH (prostate enlargement), never thinking I might be on a glide path into prostate cancer. Certainly no one ever spoke of inflammation of my prostate, and the potentially devastating impact it could have on tumor development. Nor did any mainstream physician recommend dietary changes or supplements to cool down the raging inflammation or reduce the frequency and severity of my infections.

Incredibly, it just never came up. "You might try some saw palmetto," one doctor told me. But that was the extent of it.

Instead, standard care for my prostate was limited to monitoring its enlarging size with an annual digital rectal exam, taking an annual PSA test to check for cancer, and medicating my frequent urinary tract infections with rounds of antibiotics. Looking back, it seems as if the unspoken protocol for my deteriorating prostate was to wait until I couldn't live with the symptoms any longer or the worst happens (cancer).

Both, naturally and predictably, came to pass.

I hope this will change, that clinicians will begin to put into practice the findings about the inflammation-cancer connection, and advise patients *before* the prostate gets too sick to save without a major medical intervention.

> Blog: April 7, 2008
> Today I shopped all the varieties of diapers available for guys like me in Walgreens. How did this happen?

A Coming (Baby) Boom in Prostate Cancer

A generation of boomer men is in the crosshairs for an explosion in prostate cancer, especially in the U.S. where incidence is already widespread, likely due to our high fat, high carbohydrate diets. As more boomers — those born between 1946 and 1964 — move through their 50s and 60s, the number of new cases of the disease is expected to rocket upward to 300,000 a year by 2015, according to the Prostate Cancer Foundation.[13] Today, about two million men are fighting prostate cancer; as boomer men reach the target age range for prostate cancer, by 2015 there will be another three million more men battling the disease.

Those numbers make the prostate a big business, and prostate cancer-slash-disease a highly lucrative one. *The New York Times* reported in 2009 that the average cost in the U.S. for prostate surgery was $23,000 (although I've seen costs up to $64,000), proton therapy $100,000 and targeted high-dose radiation therapy around $50,000, according the RAND Corporation data.[14]

The cost for my high-dose radiation treatment in 2008 tipped over the $100,000 mark.

These hefty pricetags for treatment go up with the rising costs of newer treatment technologies and their delivery systems. It typically costs between $125 million and $225,000 million to build new proton therapy centers, which are about the size of two football fields. Imaging costs are doubling in comparison to the overall cost of cancer care. The new vaccine, Provenge, is reportedly going for about $93,000 for treatments, and sales are expected to reach $1.5 billion a year. This is astonishing because this drug isn't a cure; it helps men with advanced cancer to extend their lives an average of four months.

PSA screens are under fire as an over-used test among the elderly with non-life threatening prostate cancer. The annual bill for the screening is about $3 billion, much of it paid by Medicare and the Veterans Administration. Add in the billions more for drugs, doctor visits and surgeries for treating BPH and prostatitis, and the prostate gland is an enormous profit center for health care providers.

Most patients, of course, never see the bill for these treatments — but we all pay for them, in the form of higher health insurance premiums. Moreover, because of the advanced age when prostate cancer afflicts most men, the cost of cutting-edge treatments like Image-Guide Radiation Therapy, da Vinci robotic surgery, and proton therapy weigh heavily on the solvency of the Medicare system. This isn't to say that these treatments aren't needed and welcomed by men in distress. They certainly are. But many elderly men have harmless, Stage 1 cancers — they don't need therapy, they're ideal watchful waiting candidates — yet they're receiving costly high-tech treatments.

With millions of boomer men moving through their "prostate years," it's no wonder overdiagnosis and over-treatment of prostate cancer are becoming topics of huge concern. Many wonder if treating older men with slow growing, non-life threatening prostate cancer with exorbitantly expensive technology may sabotage the health system all by itself.

Harvard Professor David Cutler, a Research Associate

at the National Bureau of Economic Research and a member of the Institute of Medicine, is one of them. He calls the prostate treatment problem "the poster child for overused care." In a 2010 paper for the NBER, Professor Cutler writes that while "almost all elderly men have cancer of the prostate," clinical evidence shows that the therapies are "approximately equally efficacious in men aged 65 and older" for localized prostate cancer, including watchful waiting.

In other words, *doing nothing* — except monitoring slow-growing cancer — is just as effective as surgery or radiation, but without the risk of side effects from an aggressive treatment. Professor Cutler cites new research that says the system would save "$1.7 to $3.0 billion annually" if all Medicare patients received guideline-concordant care.[15]

Of course, creating those guidelines may be trickier than finding a good screen. Still, whether older men really need expensive and aggressive treatments is something that must be sorted out with better screening and risk evaluations by physicians. Otherwise, the real financial costs of treating the prostate in an aging boomer population may implode.

The larger issue — at least in terms of human pain and suffering — is surely overtreatment, however.

In the highly-recommended book *Invasion of the Prostate Snatchers: No More Unnecessary Biopsies, Radical Treatment or Loss of Sexual Potency*, authors Ralph H.

Blum and Dr. Mark Scholz make the case that as high as 80 percent of prostatectomies done in the U.S. alone are arguably unnecessary. "Out of 50,000 radical prostatectomies performed every year in the United States alone," writes Dr. Scholz, "more than 40,000 are unnecessary. In other words, the vast majority of men with prostate cancer would have lived just as long without any operation at all. Most did not need to have their sexuality cut out."

That's a stunning statement. But the *actual* number of men being saved by aggressive treatments may be even less.

A much-heralded 2009 European study of 182,000 men reports that lives saved by prostate cancer treatment is more like 1 in every 48. For the one guy, that's great. For the other 47, not so much — as they have to live with treatment side effects.[16] Between saving that one guy and potentially maiming the lives of another 47, this is the rock and hard place — the state of the art and science in dealing with prostate cancer. It's scary.

Most urologists (who happen to be surgeons, let's not forget) continue to recommend surgery for prostate cancer treatment, even among patients with harmless Stage 1 cancers. Meanwhile, these medical experts play down the side effects. That certainly was the case for me. I was told by both my radiologist and urologist that yes there were risks, but they'd been minimized with better procedures, better technology, better this and that, blah blah blah.

It's all words until to you have to live with the outcome.

Consider all your options before deciding, and don't rush it, is all I'm saying.

Prostate Cancer:
Causes, Symptoms, Tests

The cause of prostate cancer is tough to pin down. The experts agree on many major risk factors, but the *cause*? Not yet ... or just not sure. They recognize rising PSAs in the West versus low incidence in the East. But still, the cause remains a mystery. As is the case with all cancer, science keeps striving for a consensus about what triggers the changes at the molecular level in the prostate that causes things to go so terribly wrong.

Here's a layman's explanation of what scientists at the frontier of cancer research tell us:

Prostate cancer, like all cancers, occurs when malignant cells form and spread. At a cellular level, they can see that cancer begins when cells no longer grow and divide normally. Trouble starts when new cells that the body doesn't need form and, in some situations, when old cells don't die off. Masses of tissue then come together as a growth or a tumor, which can be either benign (non-cancerous) or malignant (cancerous), the latter being potentially life threatening.

Scientists believe that when the normal cell growth process is disrupted, these malignant cells develop from changes in the DNA, which contains the genetic instructions for all types of cells. When the DNA is damaged or altered in some way — say, from chronic inflammation or even bacterial infection — the normal process for cell growth breaks down, cells begin growing out of control, tumors form, and the cancer occurs and spreads.

Interestingly, many men live with prostate cancer and don't even know it. Autopsy studies have shown that many older and even younger men who died of other diseases also had prostate cancer but exhibited no symptoms. So prostate cancer can be asymptomatic.

Autopsies also show that prostate cancer in older men is likely to coexist with BPH and prostatitis. Because the symptoms for all three are similar, physicians may initially have difficulty differentiating between the diseases.

The most common symptoms for prostate cancer, also common to BPH and prostatitis, include:

- Urinary hesitancy (delayed or slowed start of urinary stream)
- Need to urinate frequently, especially at night
- Difficulty starting or stopping urination
- Inability to feel that you have fully emptied your bladder
- Painful or burning urination or ejaculation
- Pain felt in the genital area
- Weak or interrupted flow of urine
- Difficulty having an erection
- Blood in urine or semen
- Difficulty achieving or maintaining an erection

Exams and tests for prostate cancer start with a digital rectal exam that might reveal an enlarged prostate with a hard, irregular surface that may suggest cancer. A regular PSA test can detect cancerous as well as a non-cancerous enlargement of the prostate. Your doctor can also suggest a "percent-free PSA test" that can differentiate between BPH and prostate cancer.

If all those tests suggest cancer to the physician, the prostate biopsy is commonly regarded as the only test that can identify malignant cells with certainty and confirm a cancer diagnosis. Other tests include a urine or prostatic fluid cytology that may reveal unusual cells. CT scans, a bone scan and/or a chest X-ray may be performed to see if the cancer has spread beyond the prostate gland.

None of these tests is 100 percent reliable, however. The biopsy procedure, which may snip as many as 12 pieces of tissue from the prostate, can actually miss the cancer, especially if it's a small cluster of malignant cells. If symptoms persist, the patient may have to go through additional rounds of biopsies until the cancer is found.

CT scans are performed after a diagnosis to see if the cancer is confined (localized) to the prostate or has spread. Unfortunately, today's scans are not powerful enough to see cancer at a microscopic level, so the smallest cancer cells may have escaped without notice and may reappear somewhere else years later. Doctors can tell patients the likelihood of this happening, based on their experience, grade of cancer and patient age. There's just no way of knowing for sure.

When it comes to the moment of truth — that is, deciding which treatment to pursue, if any — every patient needs to do his homework and consult multiple experts. In the early stages, doctors may recommend surgery or radiation therapy, or in older patients, they may want to monitor the cancer without recommending active treatment. If the cancer spreads beyond the prostate, it may be treated with chemotherapy, surgery (to remove the testes), or hormone therapy (to reduce testosterone levels).

Journal notes: May 2, 2009

While treatable in earlier stages of the disease, prostate cancer can be much harder to treat in more advanced stages. It's why prostate cancer is the #2 cancer killer among American men. Treatment options for prostate cancer are dictated largely by the stage of the disease, the patient's age and health, whether the cancer has just been diagnosed or has recurred, and other factors ... Every year 70,000 men require additional treatment ("salvage therapy," my doctor tells me in unsettling junkyard jargon) due to a recurrence of prostate cancer.

Risk Factors for Prostate Cancer

Age

Getting older is the greatest risk factor for prostate cancer, but certainly not the only one. According to the Prostate Cancer Research Foundation,[17] studies based on postmortem findings estimate that all men would have prostate cancer if they lived to over 100 years of age. About two-thirds of prostate cancer is diagnosed in men 65 and older. In white men with no family history of the disease, the prostate cancer risk increases significantly after the age of 50, and in African American men after the age of 40. Young men under age 30 can be diagnosed with prostate cancer, but those cases are fairly rare.

The mortality of prostate cancer increases with age as well. According to Glenn J. Bubley, associate professor of medicine at Harvard Medical School and author of *What Your Doctor May Not Tell You About Prostate Cancer* (2005), only 19 percent of all prostate cancer deaths occur before the age of 70 and approximately 42 percent after 80. But because it's common for super seniors to have competing causes of death, eliminating slow-growing prostate cancer will not necessarily prolong life, he writes. In other words, after a certain age, prostate cancer is less life threatening than other super senior diseases such as heart disease.

Family History

The risk of prostate cancer increases if you have a family history of the disease. Men who have either a father or brother diagnosed with prostate cancer have double the risk of getting it, according to the American Cancer Society.[18] The risk increases four times if you have two primary relatives diagnosed with prostate cancer. If an uncle or grandfather has the disease, the risk only goes up slightly.

The age of diagnosis is critical as well. If a father or brother is diagnosed with prostate cancer *under* the age of 60, you are more likely to carry a mutated gene that's responsible for the cancer. Your risk goes up four times because you likely possess the same faulty gene.

Race

Prostate cancer occurs in African American men about 60 percent more often than in white American men, and they are twice as likely to die from it than any other group. The incidence of prostate cancer is a little over 1 in 500 men among African Americans, which is seven times higher than the rate among Koreans, the group with the lowest rate, according to Professor Bubley.

Both Japanese and African men who live in their native countries have a low incidence of prostate cancer. Interestingly, prostate cancer rates for these groups increase sharply when they immigrate to the U.S., likely because of our Western diet. Plenty of research suggests that diets high in fat and red meats and simple sugars increase risk. The typical African American diet is thought to be relatively high in saturated fat and low in fruits and vegetables, which may offer protection.

Diet

If there's such a thing as a prostate cancer diet, you can probably sum it up in three words: *Lose the fat.* Researchers have long suspected a link between prostate cancer and a diet rich in fatty foods. The most likely culprits are meat, dairy products, and fried foods, which are high in fat, especially when compared to foods in a traditional Asian diet.

Researchers at UCLA's Jonsson Cancer Center have done studies that show a low fat, high fiber diet and regular exercise can slow prostate cancer cell growth by 30 percent.[19] Yet we continue to eat fatty foods and many doctors leave diet out of their discussion with patients. No wonder then, the rate of *prostate cancer deaths is 15 times higher* in the U.S. than in Asian countries where men traditionally eat low-fat diets. Interestingly, when Asian men immigrate to the United States and consume a typical high-fat Western diet, the incidence of prostate cancer equals the rates of Western men within a generation.

In 2008, another UCLA research team actually showed that by lowering dietary fat it helped prevent prostate cancer in mice. Most of the fat they used in the mice came from corn oil.[20] Corn oil consists mainly of omega-6 fatty acids. This is the polyunsaturated fat, often found in fried foods, that factors heavily in Western diets.

The good news is, every guy has the power to change his diet. If fat makes up 30 to 40 percent of calories in the American diet, compared to 15 percent in Japan, reducing fat consumption is a powerful step in the right direction.

Obesity
Studies on the relationship between obesity and prostate cancer have been inconsistent. However, the American Cancer Society says that obese men are at a higher risk for getting more aggressive (more dangerous) prostate cancer than men who are not considered obese. One large study[21] published in the *journal of Cancer* found that obese men increased their risk of dying from prostate cancer by 2½ times compared to men with normal weight at the time of diagnosis. Sugar intake linked to obesity may also cause inflammation in the body and prostate, setting the stage for prostate cancer development.

Inflammation
Inflammation is a sign that the immune system is doing its job in protecting us from infectious agents and injuries. However, chronic or systemic inflammation is a distinct kind of bad inflammation, what one writer referred to as "the dark side of what should be a healing process." It can occur when the tissues are continuously injured from infection or stress or irritated from pro-inflammatory foods, like those that are rapidly converted to sugar. By definition, prostatitis is a disease of inflammation and infection, and is found in a high percentage of autopsies and biopsies where prostate cancer exists.

The American Cancer Society has added inflammation to the list of key risk factors for prostate cancer. I discuss more at length the links between inflammation, diet and cancer in "The Inflammation-Cancer Connection" and "Role of Inflammation in Diet" chapters.

PART 3

THE PSA: STORM OF CONTROVERSY

To Screen or Not To Screen

Every middle-aged guy and up under a doctor's care has to deal with getting a PSA test *and* the controversy that swirls around it.

Some 30 million American men will undergo a PSA screening this year. The debate about whether the test is saving lives or leaving men to suffer needlessly as a consequence of over treatment has left many men wondering, should I screen or not screen? As always, with all things prostate, it's ultimately up to you (and your doctor) to decide.

First, some background.

The PSA test was approved in 1994 by the Food and Drug Administration (FDA) to screen for prostate cancer and detect the disease in the early stages. Before that, doctors relied on a digital rectal exam and by the time tumors could be felt, some were fairly large and in advanced stages. Now, by using a combination of the digital rectal exam and PSA test, about 90 percent of prostate cancer is found at an early and highly curable stage.

PSA stands for protein-specific antigen. The screening itself is a standard blood test, which is key to its appeal versus a rectal exam. It measures levels of prostate-specific antigens as they bind together with other substances.

PSA is a protein secreted naturally by the prostate. For the over age-50 male, a PSA test is usually carried out during an annual check-up. There is a standard rating of expected levels of prostate specific antigen. These levels increase slightly with age and that's accepted. But even a slightly elevated range is likely to warrant further investigation.

Here are the standards set by the FDA
- A measure of 4 ng/ml (nanograms per milliliter of blood) or lower is considered normal
- From 4 -10 ng/ml slightly elevated (20-30% risk)
- 10 - 20 ng/ml moderately elevated (50-75% risk)
- 20 - 30 ng/ml or above highly elevated (90% risk)

Although it's far from foolproof, the PSA test is considered the "gold standard" for early detection of prostate cancer. A negative result doesn't mean you don't have cancer, and a positive test doesn't mean you do. Infections, over-the-counter drugs and benign swelling of the prostate inflate PSA levels. Misleading results occur all the time — and therein lies the problems.

Most doctors agree that a PSA level of 4.0 ng/ml or below is considered to be safe and normal. However, some believe this level should be lowered to 2.5 ng/ml in order to detect more cases of prostate cancer. Others argue that this would exacerbate over diagnosing and over treating cancers that aren't clinically significant.

Any consistent level from 4.0 up to 10.0 is labeled suspicious and may require additional tests. Readings above

10.0 are often considered to be dangerous and may indicate that the cancer is spreading.

Many physicians now feel that the rate of increase in PSA levels — the PSA velocity — might detect life-threatening prostate cancer at a potentially curable stage, well before the 4.0 ng/ml threshold is reached.

As Predictive As 'A Coin Toss'

For years, doctors in the U.S. have routinely recommended PSA screening in men over age 50 while assuming that early diagnosis and treatment is better than standing by and doing nothing.

Generally, test results are best used as indicators of changes in PSA levels over time. If the PSA number starts going up quickly, it's usually not a good sign. If it rises more than a couple points within a year, further tests and a biopsy will likely be recommended.

On the pro-screening side of the debate, advocates argue that physicians need the information that a PSA test presents and that whether right or wrong, the PSA level is a starting place to establish a history for prostate care.

Many studies show that the PSA screening is only 60 to 70 percent accurate.[22] False positives are commonplace. Men with PSA levels in the hundreds may have no sign of cancer, and even if the antigen level is elevated, it could be due to something other than cancer. Prostatitis or an infection can elevate the level, so does aging and certain medications. Sex involving ejaculation within 48 hours of a test, strenuous exercise such as weightlifting and long stints of cycling might also skew the outcome.

With PSA levels rising from multiple factors, the National Cancer Institute[23] reports that two out of three men with high PSA readings show no cancerous cells in their prostate biopsy. Likewise, men with PSA numbers below 1 ng/ml may still have progressive cancers.

In fact, studies have shown one in five men with prostate cancer will have a normal PSA result. Perhaps that's the most frightening stat of them all — the one where the test is missing 20 percent of cancers.

So you can rightly conclude that one PSA test can be completely meaningless and that every single result needs to be confirmed. After all, the PSA tests for protein-specific antigen, not cancer.

Because of the test's uncertainty and inaccuracy, the man who discovered PSA in 1970 and revolutionized modern prostate care has turned against the test. Richard J. Albin, research professor of immunobiology and pathology at the University of Arizona College of Medicine and the president of the Robert Benjamin Albin Foundation for Cancer Research, says "… the test is hardly more effective than a coin toss."[24]

Dr. Albin goes so far as to say that the test's popularity has led to an expensive public health disaster. According to him, the PSA test is most useful *after* cancer treatment and in men with family histories of prostate cancer. Men in those categories should get tested regularly. "And if their score starts skyrocketing, it could mean cancer," Dr. Albin wrote in his article for *The New York Times*, "The Great Prostate Mistake." (May 9, 2010)

Does PSA Screening Save Lives?

Whether it's an accurate test every time or not, the PSA test is the best screen for prostate cancer that science has produced. So the next question to ask is, Does it save men's lives?

For years, most believed it did. A respected 2005 Harvard study found that men who have an annual PSA test are nearly three times less likely to die from prostate cancer than those who don't have annual screenings. The consensus was that the PSA test can detect prostate cancer long before symptoms present themselves — again, making this quick, painless procedure a simple way to discover cancer before it spreads.

Early detection from a PSA test before the cancer has spread outside the prostate also provides more treatment options and a better chance for a cure. Estimates from large, ongoing screening trials suggested that the PSA test increases the time of detection by 5 to 15 years, compared with a digital rectal exam. Therefore, it's likely that men with PSA-detected tumors will have better disease-specific survival than those who have not had the PSA test.

So there was reasonable evidence the PSA test was saving lives, until this: In 2009, a couple studies — one in Europe and the other in the United States — found that the PSA blood test saves few lives and leads to unnecessary treatments for large numbers of men. These findings, published in *The New England Journal of Medicine*,[25] cast doubt on the wisdom of the PSA test. In the European test, it was found that 48 men with prostate cancer were needlessly treated for every man whose death was prevented by the test within a decade. One in 48 lives saved — with many of those treated suffering unnecessarily the side effects of therapy — is not a very favorable endorsement of the PSA test.

Still, there are voices in the prostate world that should be listened to, and one of them is Patrick Walsh, a professor of urology and former director of the James Buchanan Brady Urological Institute at Johns Hopkins Medicine, an advocate of PSA testing. "Until an alternative exists, prostate cancer testing is the best option we have to allow men to make an informed decision. Disparaging testing does a great disservice. Because prostate cancer produces no symptoms until it's too far advanced to cure, as appropriate, men should have a PSA test and examination," he writes in his book, *Dr. Patrick Walsh's Guide to Surviving Prostate Cancer.*

Dr. Walsh makes the case that PSA testing is, indeed, saving lives. He points out that in 1988, soon after the PSA test had been introduced but before receiving FDA approval, the detection rate of advanced prostate cancer was 20 percent. By contrast, that number is only five percent today. That means medical professionals are catching more cases earlier before they advance to lethal stages. "Clearly we're doing something right," he writes. He believes the combination of early detection and better treatment is resulting in fewer men dying from prostate cancer.

Are Men Being Overtreated?

Not all prostate cancer progesses the same way. Many strains pose no threat to life and health, while others grow aggressively and are resistant to treatment. *The Wall Street Journal* (in the article "The Prostate Cancer Quandry," June 28, 2010) reported 50 percent of identified prostate cancer is too slow growing to be life threatening. That's right, *half* of all prostate cancer is not a threat — yet fear rules. As high as 90 percent of men elect to have surgery or radiation and risk the life-altering side effects. The reasons for these decisions are complex, but most guys obviously think all prostate cancer, left unchecked, is a death sentence, which is far from the truth.

The other day I'm talking to a friend whose dad, at 75, elected to have da Vinci robotic surgery for localized prostate cancer. He had a Gleason score of 6, which indicates a super slow growing cancer that's not life threatening, especially at his age: Why go through the surgery and risk the side effects of therapy? I asked.

Because, my friend explained, "my Dad wanted it out."

Get the cancer out at all costs. That's fear talking, or ignorance of the real risks. Most men don't understand not everyone needs to get rid of prostate cancer, that most ALL men will get prostate cancer if they live long enough, and that half of the prostate cancers classified so far don't have enough power to grow past the prostate gland. So they want it out. Doctors, in turn, are often obliging, and may not be educating these patients on watchful waiting as a smarter option. The medical establishment, quite frankly, is geared toward aggressive treatments.

It all starts with the PSA screen. The one we have now is so unreliable, many critics view the test as a potentially dangerous indicator. They say that even when men know they have a slow-growing cancer, they have become so anxious about prostate cancer, they want it exorcised or obliterated, despite the risk of incontinence and sexual dysfunction. These detractors also cite the cost and sometimes extreme patient discomfort of unnecessary and repeated biopsies, commonly recommended even for mildly elevated PSA levels.

So are men being overdiagnosed and overtreated? No doubt. Because of current PSA screening practices, cancer radiation centers and operating rooms are busy treating prostate cancer in men in their mid-70s and up. Legions of younger men are getting cut open and super radiated every day, risking nasty side effects for life. And in both age groups, as many as half of the men being treated have low-grade, low-risk cancers with Gleason scores of 6 and under.

Overtreatment is a serious problem — what one of my doctors called "an embarrassment to the medical profession." But until a better screen comes along to discern between the lethal and nonlethal strains of prostate cancer, the problem isn't about to go away.

Again, the weight of any decision rests on the patient. So weigh your risks. Consult with multiple physicians. Do your due diligence. Know your own cancer risks — is it considered low grade (Gleason score 6 and below) or more aggressive? Imagine, too, living your life with the side effects of the various therapies.

But be warned: overdiagnosis and overtreatment will likely continue until a better, more accurate test is devised — one in which physicians and their patients with low-grade cancer can feel more comfortable with a watchful waiting approach.

The Experts Weigh In

Unfortunately, the standards bodies who write up the clinical practice guidelines aren't all on the same page about the PSA test and whether to screen or not to screen, and when to start and stop.

Mashing all the national guidelines together, here's what I take away: Men over age 75 can skip the annual PSA screen, the cancer is generally too slow growing and treatment is unlikely to lengthen their lives. For younger men, start testing at 45 for non-risk men, age 40 for higher risk candidates.

For a little more detail, here's how the experts weigh in. Check out their websites ("Resources") for updates.

In 2009, the **American Urological Association** (AUA) updated its guidelines on prostate cancer screening for men. The AUA now recommends that men aged 40 and over who have a life expectancy of at least 10 years should be offered the PSA test to establish a baseline reading. This baseline can then help physicians diagnose, assess risk and stage cancer pre-treatment, and monitor treatment progress down the road. The AUA believes testing at the earlier age of 40 than the usually recommended 50 "may allow for earlier detection of curable cancer."

The **American Cancer Society** (ACS) seems more

wishy-washy on the subject, because the benefits of the test, they say, are "unclear or unproven." They recommend that men make "an informed decision" with their doctor about whether to be tested for prostate cancer. The ACS does not support routine testing for prostate cancer. Instead, it recommends patients discuss the benefits and drawbacks of the PSA test at age 50 for most men and 45 for high-risk patients. High-risk men include African Americans, plus fathers, brothers or sons who have been diagnosed with prostate cancer.

The **U.S. Preventive Services Task Force** (USPSTF) says the evidence is "insufficient" and the benefits "slim to none" to recommend for or against routine screening for prostate cancer. In its 2008 upgraded guidelines, the members recommended *against* routine screening in men age 75 years or older.

The **Prostate Cancer Foundation** favors screening, and early, for high-risk patients. They say that age 40 is a reasonable time to start to screen those men with a genetic disposition or who are African American. For otherwise healthy men at high risk, 40 to 45 is reasonable. They don't provide guidelines for men at average risk, but recommend starting testing at age 50 in order to create a proactive prostate health plan.

Most experts continue to believe early detection with the PSA test is the smart way to go, at least until new tests are perfected. So talk to your doctor.

Despite the risk of overtreatment, I fall on the side of regular PSA screening, and the common sense wisdom of Dr. Peter Carroll, Chair of the American Urological Association panel on prostate testing guidelines. In the release of the AUA's 2009 guidelines, he said, "Prostate cancer comes in many forms, some aggressive and some not. But the bottom line about prostate cancer testing is that we cannot counsel patients about next steps for cancer that we do not know exist."

J. Brantley Thrasher, M.D., chairman of urology at the University of Kansas Medical Center in Kansas City, Kansas, and spokesman for the American Urological Association, agreed. "(Prostate cancer) is a silent killer. So most men with a nodule or elevated PSA aren't going to know it ... (The PSA test) is an imperfect marker, but it's the best we've got."[26]

What Elevates and Lowers Your PSA?

Getting a reliable PSA test can seem like a crapshoot after reading about its many flaws. But it's right much of the time, just not all the time. So confirm all results. Be aware that the most mundane or unsuspecting activities can influence your PSA level. In part because of the many factors that can artificially raise or lower a PSA level, most physicians recommend that a PSA should be repeated, often several times before a biopsy. Some physicians will prescribe antibiotics for three to six weeks if they find evidence or a history of prostate infection.

First, things that might *elevate* your test results:
- Sex. Doctors generally recommend men should abstain from sex at least two days prior to testing Studies show that ejaculation within that period

before a PSA test may increase PSA levels in the blood.

- Stimulation of the prostate from rigorous physical activity. Activities like a prostate massage or a long bike ride could elevate PSA levels.
- Inflammation of the prostate gland. Prostate problems, such as BPH or prostatitis, can inflate PSA levels.
- Infections of the prostate. They may cause PSA levels to rise, even as an infection can produce no symptoms.
- A man with a larger than average prostate may have a higher than normal PSA reading, even if his prostate is healthy. A larger prostate produces more PSA into the blood.
- Digital rectal exams and biopsies of the prostate may cause PSA levels to rise. It should be noted that an increase in PSA caused by a DRE is not thought to be significant enough to produce a false-positive result. On the other hand, a biopsy could elevate PSA levels for as long as four weeks.
- Age alone can increase PSA levels. The older a man gets, the likelier his PSA will rise, yet it may mean nothing. For instance, a man might have a PSA reading of 5.5 ng/ml at age 70, and not have cancer, yet that same score in a 50-something male would raise concern.

What can *lower* your PSA levels?

- Certain medications used to control urinary problems from BPH and prostatitis — such as finasteride (the hair growth medication Propecia) or dustasteride (prescribed for BPH, called Avodart), which are prescription medications, or saw palmetto, an over-the-counter herbal remedy — can lower PSA levels by as much as 50 percent.
- Research published in *Cancer*[27] shows that men who use common painkillers such as nonsteroidal anti-inflammatory drugs (NSAIDs) and aspirin on a regular basis had PSA levels that were about 10 percent lower than the men who did not use them.

Predicting Risk and Avoiding Unnecessary Biopsies

PSA Velocity

PSA velocity measures how fast a man's PSA level increases from year to year. It can be a valuable predictor of prostate cancer — not only to determine if you have it now, but if you might develop life-threatening prostate cancer many years from now. Many experts regard PSA velocity as a more powerful predictor of prostate cancer than the PSA test itself.

Experts believe that men with rapidly rising PSA, rather than a slow rising PSA, face greater risk for aggressive disease and, therefore, in need of treatment. For anyone recently diagnosed who is considering watchful waiting, this is a good measurement to factor into your decision-making.

Johns Hopkins Research has done exceptional work in this area. According to a study they did with National Institute of Health, an increase in PSA level of more than 0.75 ng/ml per year in men with PSA levels between 4 to 10 ng/ml is an early predictor of prostate cancer.[28]

A rapid rise in one year suggests the presence of cancer. This happened to me. My PSA level soared from 1 ng/ml to 6.6 ng/ml within 12 months. That increase alarmed my urologist to the presence of an "aggressive" cancer, which proved to be on the money after my biopsy and the pathology report.

Percent-Free PSA

Biopsies can be painful and should be avoided whenever possible, that's a given. They may have severe complications, among them infections and hemorrhaging, or worse. A study at the University of California, San Diego, shows that stimulating cancerous tissue through prostate biopsies may actually promote the spread of the cancer.

However, if your PSA test and digital rectal exam suggest cancer, then your doctor will recommend a biopsy in order to confirm a cancer diagnosis and identify the grade of cancer. It's the only way to know for sure. You need to know what a biopsy reveals before deciding on a treatment, but keep this in mind: *Less than 1 percent of the prostate tissue is examined in each biopsy, which leaves more than 99 percent of the gland unexamined.*

This explains why biopsies can come back negative, yet cancer is still present. Only 29 percent of cancer cases are detected in the first biopsy.[29]

So what happens if the biopsy shows no cancer and the PSA level remains elevated? Cancer may still be indicated yet the biopsy didn't find it. Now what?

Fortunately, the percent-free PSA test can indicate to your physician whether another biopsy is absolutely necessary (perhaps there's another reason the PSA is elevated). What's more, the percent-free PSA can also be a safeguard against a biopsy that may *miss* the cancer.

Let me explain: Prostate-specific antigen floats in the blood in two forms — attached (or bound) to blood proteins and unattached (or unbound) to blood proteins. The percent-free PSA test measures the proportion of unattached PSA to the total PSA in the blood sample.

What does that mean? Well, the percentage of percent-free PSA is lower in men who have prostate cancer than in men who do not. According to American Cancer Society, men with percent-free PSA at 7 percent or lower — meaning 7 percent is floating freely and unattached to blood proteins — prostate cancer is likely and the patient should undergo a biopsy.

Many doctors advise that men "consider" a biopsy if the level of free and unbounded PSA is between 7 percent and 25 percent, although the 25 percent threshold is not agreed upon by all doctors. A high free PSA — above 25 percent — usually indicates BPH (benign prostate hyperplasia) and not cancer.

My urologist had me take a percent-free PSA before my first biopsy. It was an 8, indicating a biopsy should be recommended.

Using these cutoffs can help doctors detect prostate cancer with more certainty than a single, straightforward PSA test. Plus, the initial PSA test is generally not strong evidence of prostate cancer. So the follow-up free PSA test is usually performed if the original results are suspicious.

The percent-free PSA test helps a physician decide if the patient should have a prostate biopsy, especially if the regular PSA results are in the borderline range — between 4 and 10 ng/ml of blood.

While the free PSA test can spare some men unnecessary biopsies, conversely, it can act as a safety net for patients who have a suspicious PSA level but their biopsies come back negative (no found cancer). For instance, if the biopsy comes back negative with no found cancer but the free PSA remains low, a repeat biopsy is in order. That would suggest that the biopsy might have missed the cancer.

> ### Journal: March 8, 2010
> (Almost two years after diagnosis and therapy)
>
> My PSA bounce arrived!... My PSA had been steadily dropping over 18 months since the radiation treatment ended, to 0.9 ng/ml, which is normal for someone with a prostate. Then three months ago, it suddenly jumped to 1.9 ng/ml — the phenomena called the "PSA bounce." I knew it might be coming, it happens to lots of guys — but knowing doesn't relieve the anxiety of wondering, Is can cancer coming back? What then? But today my level dropped to 1.0 ... normal again. Interestingly, the sudden rise may be worth the short-term anxiety. I read a study that said men with PSA bounces have a reduced risk of the cancer returning.

PART 4

EATING FOR A HEALTHY PROSTATE

Role of Inflammation in Diet

Diet has long been a suspected culprit of prostate cancer. No question, age and genetics are key risk factors that predispose men to prostate maladies. But what we put in our mouths over time may be the trigger that sets prostate diseases, and cancer, in motion. The World Health Organization[30] believes that one-third of all cancers might be avoided by dietary changes alone.

One of the more compelling arguments targeting diet's role in prostate health is the prevalence of prostate cancer in Western versus Asian countries. In Western countries, there is a striking 30 to 50 times greater incidence of prostate cancer than in Asia, according to the National Health Institute (www.nih.gov). Yet when Asian men migrate to Western countries and adopt a Western lifestyle and diet, their prostate cancer incidence rises to match Western men within a generation. Likewise, African American men have the highest prostate cancer risk in the world, yet prostate cancer incidence is very low in Africa.

The Western diet — high in saturated fat, sugar and red meat, and low in fiber, fruits and vegetables — has been proven to lead directly to chronic low-level inflammation. This has been repeatedly linked to the development of prostate cancer. Hence, the Western diet — perhaps in conjunction with heredity factors — factors into pro-inflammatory conditions that lead to prostate cancer.

Americans have been eating a high-fat, high-carbohydrate diet for decades. One of worst culprits is sugar. When you raise your blood sugar level, you cause an insulin response in the body that, in turn, produces inflammation on the cellular level. The more insulin you trigger with sugar, the greater the levels of inflammation throughout the body, including the prostate. At the Duke Prostate Center, researchers have shown that insulin contributes to the growth and proliferation of prostate cancer. In the bodies of mice, they also report a diet devoid of carbohydrates actually lowers serum insulin levels, resulting in the slowing of tumor growth.[31]

Despite mounting research, the inflammation-cancer connection, discussed earlier, is still not a common topic of discussion between prostate patients and the mainstream physicians who are treating them. Yet many leading scientists digging into the causes of prostate disease and cancer have been publishing plenty of research over the last decade on how diet, inflammation and cancer are linked.

So again, it's up to men to do their own homework on how to remedy an unhealthy prostate, or perhaps even prevent the worst case scenario of prostate cancer by adopting an anti-inflammatory diet as they have in Asian countries.

Anthony J. Sattilaro, M.D., did his homework. He was president of Methodist Hospital in Philadelphia when he was diagnosed with prostate cancer. In his best-selling book, *Recalled by Life*, he describes how he began following a "macrobiotic" diet, rich in traditional Asian foods, including plenty of rice and vegetables. Far outliving his initial grave prognosis, the diet made him one of the more famous advocates for the use of diet, herbs and vitamins to fight cancer.

My point is this: While you may not have any control over your gene pool, you certainly can control the pro-inflammatory foods you eat. There are many anti-inflammatory diets on the market today, including the Mediterranean diet. Here are some basic guidelines to follow if you want to create your own.

> **Journal: March 8, 2010**
> A steady diet of red meat and dairy cheese is a terrible combo for prostate health. In countries where they're not a mainstay in the diet or even largely absent, so is prostate cancer, at least in the way we experience it. So the quintessential anti-prostate meal: a fat ol' cheeseburger with greasy fries.

Anti-Inflammation Diet: The Basics

Avoid low starches and other simple sugars — The cornerstone of any anti-inflammation diet is regulating blood sugar. Low starches and simple sugars elevate insulin and glucose levels, which exacerbate inflammatory conditions. Avoid simple carbohydrates or high glycemic index foods like potatoes, any kind of rice, all corn, cakes, pastries, pies, all pastas such as macaroni, spaghetti, noodles, or crackers, chips and tortillas. (Yes, unfortunately, the good stuff.)

Many people don't realize pro-inflammatory foods may appear as a nutritious and tasty choice, but once digested, rapidly convert into sugar in the body. Examples: potatoes, bananas, fruit juices, processed cereals, breads, rice and pasta. All of these high-glycemic foods cause blood sugar to rapidly rise, and thus trigger an increase in insulin and inflammation in the cells.

No high fructose corn syrup — The American diet is awash in large amounts of high fructose corn syrup (what may soon be renamed "corn sugar"), replacing sucrose in most soft drinks, candies and processed foods. This inexpensive and processed sugar is associated with development of the insulin resistance syndrome. Read the label for corn syrup, fructose or high fructose corn syrup. Not only are they found in the usual suspects like soft drinks and snacks, but also in many meal replacement bars and diet drinks.

Eat high ratio of omega-3 to omega-6 fats — This one suddenly got murky. Multiple studies over the last decade have found a diet rich in inflammation-lowering omega-3 reduces the risk of aggressive prostate cancer. One study (published in *Clinical Cancer Research*, April 2009) found men who ate at least one serving of fatty fish per week reduced their risk of prostate cancer by a whopping 63 percent when compared to men who never ate this type of fish. The researchers noted that omega-3 fatty acids also protect against heart disease by targeting inflammation. Omega-3 foods contain essential fatty acids, found in generous amounts in salmon.

Yet along comes a new nationwide study involving more than 3,400 men that claims just the opposite — that omega-3 actually increases the risk of developing aggressive, high grade prostate cancer by two-and-a-half times. This has turned the thinking about omega-3 upside down.

Predictably, many experts have questioned the study, published by researchers at Fred Hutchinson Cancer Research Center in the *American Journal of Epidemiology* (April 2011). They point out that subjects also took finasteride (Propecia and Proscar), and that drug may have influenced the interactions with dietary fats.

Other experts have argued that the most important factor in lowering the risk of prostate cancer is the *balance* between omega-3 and omega-6 fatty acids. Most Western diets have ratios of omega-6 to omega-3 in excess of 10 to 1, some much higher at 30 to 1. The ideal balance is believed to be 4 to 1 or lower, according to research from the Center of Genetics (*Nutrition and Health*, May 2002). The lower the ratio, the higher the anti-inflammatory properties in the body.

Again, accumulating evidence shows that chronic inflammation can promote all stages of tumor development, including DNA damage, leading to cancer.

Stay turned as this one gets sorted out in future studies.

No trans fats — Trans fats are used by the food industry to extend shelf life and flavor, but all of them are pro-inflammatory and boost cancer risk. In many areas of food processing, trans fats have taken the place of healthier natural solid fats and liquid oils. Trans fats can effectively double the risk of non-aggressive prostate cancer tumors, according to a Harvard study that followed almost 15,000 men over 13 years. This fat is found in processed or fast foods, especially fried foods.

Take probiotics — This is the good bacteria that lines your gut and helps with many bodily functions in the digestive system, like lowering intestinal pH, controlling growth of pathogens, and preventing bad bacteria from taking over your intestinal walls. Potential benefits range from managing lactose intolerance to lowering cholesterol, lowering blood pressure, preventing colon cancer, improving immune function and preventing infections. Probiotics are also vitally important in reducing inflammation and offer anti-cancer potential. Nutritionists advise that it's crucial for anyone on antibiotics — often prescribed for prostatitis — to take probiotic supplements to keep their digestive system in balance.

Low saturated fats — You can reduce inflammation in the body by reducing the amount saturated fats you ingest. Meat and dairy products are high in saturated fat. Cow's milk products contain a protein that causes chronic inflammation and should be avoided. Eat either lean cuts of organic meats, chicken, turkey or fish. Butter is a saturated fat, but when eaten in small amounts like one teaspoon, it usually burns off as energy and is not stored as fat in the body.

More fruit and vegetable antioxidants — Fruits and

vegetables, as well as tea and wine, are high in inflammation-reducing antioxidants, especially onions, garlic, peppers and dark leafy greens, as well as inflammation-fighting carotenoids, like vitamin K and vitamin E. Tip: The more colorful your natural plant foods, the richer the food tends to be in antioxidants.

Drink coffee — A couple major Harvard studies, the first in 2009 and a second in 2011, showed that men who drank six or more cups of coffee a day were 60 percent less likely to develop deadly metastatic prostate cancer than men who drank no coffee. A similar reduction was shown with decaffeinated coffee drinkers. One to three cups cut the risk of lethal prostate cancer by 30 percent. Coffee and chocolate both contain anti-inflammatory antioxidants and minerals that are associated with reducing the prostate cancer risk.

Green tea — Consumption of green tea has long been a favorite anti-inflammatory antioxidant among holistic healers. Apparently, they are right. In 2009, a study published in Cancer Prevention Research showed that men with prostate cancer who drank green tea showed a significant reduction in certain serum markers — including protein-specific antigen — which are predictive of prostate cancer progression.

Researchers in China have also found that the risk of prostate cancer declined with green tea consumption. Green tea contains antioxidants, which destroy free radicals produced when our bodies convert food to energy. Left unchecked, free radicals can lead to cell and DNA damage, putting people at greater risk of cancer and other diseases.

Prostate-Friendly, Anti-Inflammatory Supplements

Antibiotics for prostatitis and pharmaceuticals to treat BPH and over-active bladder syndrome are conventional or "standard" therapies to promote easier urination. However, herbal and homeopathic approaches to prostate health may offer more natural remedies with fewer harmful side effects. In Europe and other countries, physicians seem more open to natural prostate supplements than American doctors and widely prescribe them. The one herbal exception might be saw palmetto, which is increasingly recommended by U.S. physicians, especially to treat BPH.

The issue for mainstream U.S. physicians seems to be a lack of hard-core science that supports recommending many herbal remedies. You might find a more receptive ear by consulting a nutritionist, or perhaps an alternative medical practitioner or even an acupuncturist. These professionals can help you find supplements that work best for you.

While supplements can play an important role in prostate health, they shouldn't be taken mindlessly. In addition to talking with a medical expert, you want to maximize safety, therapeutic dosage, and, efficacy by always sourcing your supplements from a reputable company. In the unregulated supplements industry, quality versus crap is a huge issue... tread wisely.

Saw palmetto — Of the three herbs best known for treating prostate disease (saw palmetto, nettle root and pygeum africanum), saw palmetto is the best studied. Studies have suggested that saw palmetto is effective in treating BPH by inhibiting the conversion of testosterone to dihydrotestosterone, which is believed to enlarge the prostate. The history of saw palmetto traces back 12,000 years to Florida aborigines and later the Seminole Indians who used it to treat impotence, inflammation of the prostate and low libido.

Beta-sitosterol — This plant sterol is found in small quantities in pecans, saw palmetto, avocados, pumpkin seeds, wheat germ, soybeans and pygeum africanum. But it is now marketed in highly concentrated forms as a supplement, usually in combination with saw palmetto. Beta-sitosterol is said to be about 3000 times more potent than saw palmetto. But like saw palmetto, the jury is still out on the efficacy on men with BPH and prostatitis. However, several months before my cancer diagnosis, I started taking it for for the first time and my symptoms for BPH and chronic prostatitis began to disappear significantly after four weeks. Apparently, beta-sitosterol is also used in Europe as a supplement in the treatment of both prostate cancer and breast cancer.

Pygeum africanum — This anti-inflammatory herb comes from an African evergreen tree. By reducing the hormone prolactin in the body, it lowers both the uptake and accumulation of testosterone in the prostate. European doctors, who have widely prescribed pygeum africanum for decades, believe it can also helpful in increasing urine flow and even improving sexual performance.

Nettle root — Like saw palmetto, nettle root (also known as stinging nettle) has anti-inflammatory properties that inhibit the enzyme involved with the conversion of testosterone to dihydrotestosterone. In excess, dihydrotestosterone causes pathological prostate growth. Researchers have found that the size of the prostate gland decreases after taking the extract for 12 weeks, and with the shrinkage, a decrease in frequency by as much as 50 percent.

Epilobium parviflorum — This herb has been shown to have an anti-inflammation and healing effect on chronic and acute inflammation of the prostate and BPH. Many physicians recommend epilobium parviflorum for all men over the age of 50 as a way to prevent and maintain not only prostate health but a healthy bladder as well.

> Journal: January 21, 2009
> (Eight months after radiation treatment)
> I had another digital exam today — how many is that?
> 20 or 30? Only this time I got a result I hadn't heard for
> almost 10 years. Dr. WS described my prostate as
> "smooth, supple and small" ... that may've described
> the apparatus too, but whatever ... everything checks
> out, my PSA is 1.4, and still dropping — I'm cancer free,
> as best as anyone can tell. I'll take it....

PART 5

PSA RISING?... WELL, IT'S A JOURNEY

Only days after publishing the first edition of *The Prostate Storm*, I was reminded prostate cancer is a journey — an unending journey, an ultramarathon. That day I get a call from my urologist's office. The nurse tells me the doctor wants to see me "immediately" about my latest PSA level.

My alarm bells going off, I naturally ask what the number was. I had just taken my tenth follow-up PSA test after high-dose radiation treatment 28 months earlier, but I didn't know the result. The nurse tells me 1.5 (ng/ml), which initially was a relief, but I realized too it had risen from a nadir of 0.9 to 1.3 and now 1.5 in just six months.

I wasn't sure what a little bump up like that meant. A year ago I had experienced a full point jump, the phantom "bounce" which happens to a lot of guys who have radiation therapy; it settled back to the nadir within three months.

No harm, no foul.

But like most guys with prostate cancer, I also had a history of BPH and prostatitis, which can influence PSA levels, so my initial reaction to this latest bump was not to worry. A small rise could be attributable to lots of things, including sex or even strenuous exercise. So I asked the nurse to have the urologist to please call me, but she explained the doctor didn't make phone calls to patients "otherwise he'd be doing that all the time." She insisted Dr. JM wanted to see me "as soon as possible" — which, she said, would have to be next Friday, a full week away.

Huh? Doctor raises my anxiety level to Defcon 5, he won't call me, and he won't see me for seven days—what kind of patient care is that? Is that how the "cancer may be returning" message is delivered?

I asked again, "Would you please have him call me," and she said very nicely she would talk to the doctor but no guarantees. Great. Meanwhile, I'll let my imagination go wild for a week, thank you very much …

Surprisingly, a day later, the urologist does call me, though obviously irritated that he's on the phone with me instead of delivering a digital rectal exam. But he insists, "I need to check you out right away because three rises in a row could indicate another biopsy and radiation failure" but adds that I should not worry because I have options for failed radiation, "like freezing the cancer …"

What f*ing cancer? I'm in a state of shock, I'm cancer free. Or thought I was. One minute I'm a prostate cancer survivor, the nightmare of biopsies and confusing treatment choices and massive radiation two-and-a-half years ago behind me — the next moment, out of the blue, I'm confronting "radiation failure" and "another biopsy" and uncertain outcomes.

In a blink it seems, I'm staring into the blunt junkyard language of a prostate cancer still stalking me: Salvage therapy.

Over and over again in *The Prostate Storm*, I drum the point that if you catch most types of prostate cancer earlier enough with PSA testing, the cure rate is the absolute best in the cancer business — around 95 percent. But for that 1-in-20 guy, those stats provide little solace. For that guy, he eventually gets the word the cancer is back. Was that me? Am I that stat?

We can all worry about being that guy who lost the statistical lottery, but I didn't really think that would be me. Nobody does, especially with such favorable odds, until I heard "radiation failure" from Dr. JM — and even then I wasn't buying it.

"Any time you have three rises, it suggests radiation failure," he says to me, flatly.

"And you think these two incremental rises (from .9 to 1.3 to 1.5) are significant?"

"Yes."

Trying to sort this out, I'm fully aware of my troubled history with prostatitis and BPH, both diseases of the prostate, that can drive up PSA levels. Since the radiation treatment, I haven't experienced any pronounced symptoms, but still — I had a history. The PSA test is also influenced by so many arbitrary things, besides being an unreliable indicator of cancer. Maybe something is artificially elevating the PSA level, I'm thinking.

"Why can't I just have another PSA is three months and then see where I'm at?" I ask.

"What, are you trying to be a urologist?" he snaps at me, increasingly agitated with this phone call and my questions. "I need you to come in so I can do the research." The research? The only research he could do is a DRE, a feeling around for any new hardness on the surface of the prostate.

Granted, I probably should've followed the doctors orders and gone to the appointment for the DRE. But I didn't. Instead, I talked with three other doctors, including another urologist, to see how worried I should be about the two incremental rises. All of them told me not to worry, that the PSA can bounce around at this level.

"Plus you do have a history with prostatitis," my family physician said. Sit tight, they all advised me, and have another PSA in three months and take it from there. But if it rises over 2 ng/ml, they said that I should take the pattern serious and be prepared that a biopsy may be recommended.

While their advice was somewhat of a relief, my urologist's premature warning had served a purpose: He made me realize that despite an aggressive treatment, I still lived in the cancer world, I'd never left it, and I never would. Whether the trend of a couple rising PSAs is not my friend, or an inconsequential blip, I shouldn't assume anything, good or bad.

Several days later, I received a letter from the urologist telling me that I had a "medical situation that needed immediate care" but that his practice would no longer provide that care.

In other words, I was fired as a patient.

Whatever. The guy was a jerk. The conversation should've gone something like, "Steve, the PSA can bounce around but let's just be conservative because of the two rises, let me examine you, and then we'll have a PSA in three months and take it from there. If it gets over 2.0 ng/ml, we may need to consider a biopsy. Hopefully, it's nothing."

I could've lived with that. He would have put me on notice, without undue alarm, got the DRE and let me know we're watching the PSA closely now. I would've gone in and felt like my doctor was being typically conservative but looking out for me.

Instead, he just scared the crap out of me.

For two days after our conversation, I was a wreck, more so than when I got the original cancer diagnosis. Because now I knew more. I did radiation, and survived the treatment and, worse for me, the six-month recovery suffering through overactive bladder syndrome, nasty rectal burn, long bouts with hemorrhoids and the onset of mild erectile dysfunction.

I thought I'd moved to the other side of these miseries, but I was mistaken. What I knew about salvage therapy is that the collateral damage from a second treatment can be rough. For starters, they won't do surgery to radiation patients. Nor will they do more high-dose radiation. My options were freezing the prostate or hormone therapy, or some combination… in any event, the side effects of a second major treatment are not pleasant to think about.

I kept telling myself, let's not get too far ahead of the facts. I need another PSA test, and another after that. I need to see if a rising PSA is a pattern, or an anomaly, and I may have to do that forever until they discover a better and more predictive screen. But yeah, if my PSA keeps rising, I'll have to start looking into my options all over again.

Starting with a new urologist.

As with all people who've been diagnosed with cancer, you live with it long after treatment. Recurrence is always a possibility, so you need good and caring doctors whom you can trust and feel comfortable with. Even though my urologist may've had a horrible bedside manner on the phone and I may've not been the best patient, he did shake me out of a false sense of being done with the cancer.

Three months later, my PSA dropped to 1.0 ng/ml, followed by another low number the next quarter. So something had temporary aggravated my prostate, causing the bump up. Most likely a recurring bout with prostatitis, but I don't know for sure. I only know that the trend line up had been broken and I didn't have to sweat about another biopsy or salvage therapy, at least not yet.

Still, while my urologist is now history, he did contribute something invaluable to my post-treatment care and I should probably send him a *Thank You* note and an explanation: He reminded me, inartfully as it was, that a run with prostate cancer has no finish line. We continue to monitor it regularly, we take a deep breath before results come in, and we don't take anything for granted. Or at least we shouldn't.

Cancer is a journey, and once you get on line, you can never get off.

The Prostate Storm

⯈ A Final Word

Gentlemen, get your PSA test annually, starting at age 40 (earlier than recommended, especially if it's in the family) or 45 at the latest. Catching it early means that most prostate cancer, but not all unfortunately, will be more of an inconvenience than a game-changer.

Hopefully, in the near future, we will have a more reliable screen, likely a gene test, that will differentiate between deadly metastatic prostate cancer and the non-lethal variety. That will eliminate about half of the radiation and surgical treatments that are unnecessary and may be doing more harm than good. Remember, all guys who live long enough will get prostate cancer, but not all of it needs to be aggressively treated. So know your cancer risks before choosing any course of therapy.

And always eat for a healthy prostate. Among the high risk factors, you can't control aging and genetics, but you can control your diet. Lose the fat, cut the sugar. You may even spend less time in the bathroom.

Finally, support prostate cancer research — and help find a cure to spare our sons.

ACKNOWLEDGMENTS

This book is based almost entirely on my experience with prostate cancer, research I dug up on the Internet, books I read in sorting through the maze of information about prostate disease and treatment options, and conversations with physicians. I am deeply indebted to the men and women who posted comments about their own experiences on the countless Internet discussion forums that I browsed during the weeks before and shortly after my diagnosis. To me, they are the foot soldiers in the trenches, having real and intimate experiences with the promises of modern technology. I want to thank all of those Bobs and Jims and Carols and Freds who, in their anonymity, gave me a glimpse into the fear, confusion and blind faith that exists in the world of faltering prostates.

I want to thank Dr. Mark Chelmowski and Dr. Michael Vernacchio, both of whom were very generous with their time to answer my questions and give my manuscript a careful read for any wrong-headed medical statements. While reviewing the material, they approached the book with fair and open minds, and their insights were invaluable. Even though the book challenges some conventional wisdom regarding mainstream medicine's approach to prostate issues, I needed real physicians looking over my shoulder. I am grateful to both of them.

Barbara McNichol, my editor in Tuscon, Arizona, provided excellent editing and extraordinary sensitivity to the subject matter. Chris O'Byrne, of Red Willow Publishing (www.redwillowpublishing.com), provided invaluable guidance and support in getting *The Prostate Storm* ready for publication and distributed. My thanks to both of you.

The American Cancer Society, the Prostate Cancer Foundation and the Livestrong Foundation, American Urological Association Foundation, National Cancer Institute, National Prostate Cancer Coalition and the Prostate Net were invaluable sources of information on the Internet. I recommend anyone going through any prostate problems, including cancer, take a careful look at the websites of these organizations. Endless resources are at your fingertips.

I cannot say enough about the extraordinary research produced by Johns Hopkins Medical Research at the James Buchanan Brady Urological Institute in Baltimore, Maryland. (http.//urology.jhu.edu/index.html). I downloaded many of their white papers and research to gain insight and background for the medical discussions within the book, especially those focused on inflammation as a common link between prostate disease, prostate cancer and diet. I hope their important work and breakthrough research will inform doctors at the clinical level sooner rather than later.

I ran across many incredible first-person blogs written by people documenting their own experiences with prostate cancer. One of the best is Dana Jennings for *The New York Times*. He's a fabulous writer and reporter and walks you through his experience of having more advanced prostate cancer, and he does it with humor and a reporter's eye. (http://well.blogs.nytimes.com/author/dana-jennings)

He provided many insights for this book.

The following books and ebooks were useful points of reference and valued sources for statistics and quotes, and would make for excellent reading: *Dr. Patrick Walsh's Guide to Surviving Prostate Cancer* by Patrick Walsh, M.D., *What Your Doctor May Not Tell You About Prostate Cancer* by Glenn J. Bubley, M.D., *Prostate Health in 90 days without drugs or surgery* and *Prostatitis: The 60-Day Cure* by Dr. Larry Clapp, *The Inflammation Syndrome* by Jack Challem, *The Perricone Prescription* by Nicholas Perricone, M.D., *Seven Keys to Treating Prostate Cancer* by Jacek L. Mostwin, M.D. of Johns Hopkins Medicine, *All About the Prostate* by Ben Org, and *Men at Risk, a Rush to Judgment* by Dr. Ronald Wheeler; *Invasion of the Prostate Snatchers: No More Unnecessary Biopsies, Radical Treatment or Loss of Sexual Potency* by Mark Scholz, M.D., and Ralph Blum; and *Recalled by Life* by Anthony J. Sattilaro, M.D.

Thanks, too, to my mom and her husband, Ed Smith, who were the first to read my manuscript during a vacation to Hawaii. For taking time out between luaus and for their first encouraging reviews, I am very grateful.

My son, Nick, was an unwitting inspiration in having me face prostate cancer with the same unflappable cool I saw him exhibit as a pitcher on his high school baseball team. No matter how adverse the situation behind him, he never seemed affected, never let down, never succumbed to the pressure. He always stayed focused on the next pitch at hand and executed. One pitch at a time. Staying in the moment. No panic. When the chips were down, that's what

I tried to do too.

Finally, my wife, Lorraine, lived through this book from the anxiety leading up to the diagnosis, to the genesis of the blog that chronicled my prostate cancer experience, to dealing with cancer and writing and publishing this book. She is the one who convinced me to turn the blog into a book in the first place.

Lorraine is a creative soul and exceptionally gifted jewelry maker and graphic designer, who currently works as the art director for a pair of stylish regional magazines. So she created the gorgeous cover design and laid out the interior pages for me. This book exists — and is infinitely richer — because of her.

ENDNOTES

1 Kolata, Results Unproven, Robotic Surgery Wins Converts, *The New York Times*, February 13, 2010
2 *The Lancelot Oncology,* (May 2010)
3 www.cancer.org
4 ibid
5 Johns Hopkins Health Alerts, http://www.johnshopkinshealthalerts. com/symptoms_remedies/prostate_cancer/88-1.html
6 Prostate Cancer – Biology, Diagnosis, Pathology, Staging, and Natural History, Emedicine, http://emedicine.medscape.com/ article/458011-overview
7 Is BPH an Immune Disease? *European Urology*, Dec. 11, 2006
8 What Does Inflammation Have to Do With Cancer, *Prostate Cancer Discovery*, http://urology.jhu.edu
9 Johns Hopkins Health Alerts, Prostate Disorders – The Inflammation-Prostate Cancer Link, January 11, 2007.
10 Diagnosis of prostatic inflammation, *Urology*, www.goldjournal.*net*
11 The results were published in *New England Journal of Medicine*, April 1, 2009.
12 www.cancerhelp.org.uk
13 www.pcf.org
14 Leonhardt, In Health Reform, a Cancer Offers Acid Test, July 2009
15 National Bureau of Economic Research, October 28, 2010
16 Schroeder, M.D., et al, Screening and Prostate-Cancer Mortality in a Randomized European Study, *New England Journal of Medicine*, March 26, 2009
17 www.pcf.org
18 www.cancer.org
19 Diet, Exercise Slow Prostate Cancer As Much As 30%, *UniSci*, www.unisci.com/stories/20013/9011013.htm
20 Eating less fat may prevent prostate cancer, UCLA Newsroom, http://newsroom.ucla.edu
21 journal of Cancer, March 15, 2007
22 Hoffman, MD, Screening for prostate cancer, May 3, 2010,
23 National Cancer Institute, www.cancer.gov/cancertopics, reference PSA estimates
24 Richard Albin, The Great Prostate Mistake, *The New York Times*, March 9, 2010
25 Schroeder, M.D., et al, Screening and Prostate-Cancer Mortality in a Randomized European Study, *New England Journal of Medicine*, March 26, 2009
26 *FDA Consumer*, May-June 2006
27 *Cancer* 2008

28 Understanding PSA, www.johnshopkinshealthalerts.com
29 *Journal of Urology* 2002
30 www.who.int
31 *Cancer Prevention Research*, May 26, 2009

Here's a partial listing of additional research and articles I referenced in various medical journals via web searches for the book.

• Guided Radiation Therapy for Prostate Cancer Prevents Damage to Surrounding Organs, Oregon Health and Science University, October 29, 2007, http://www.physorg.com/news112801420.html
• Men with Prostate Cancer Avoid Radiation Due to Misconceptions, American Cancer Society for Therapeutic Radiology and Oncology, http://www.sciencedaily.com/releases/2006/11/061105211730, November 6, 2006
• Schaeffer AJ, Wendel EF, Dunn JK, et al. Prevalence and Significance of Prostatic Inflammation,: *Journal of Urology*, Vol. 125, 1981
• Nelson WG, DeMarzo AM, DeWeese TL, et al, The Role of Inflammation in the Pathogenesis of Prostate Cancer, *Journal of Urology*, Vol. 172, 2004
• Smith GR and Missailidis S, Inflammation and the AT1 and AT2 receptors, Cancer, *Journal of Inflammation*, Vol.1, 2004
• Coussens LM and Werb Z, Inflammation and Cancer, *Nature*, Vol. 420, 2002
• Balkwill F and Mantovani A, Inflammation and Cancer: Back to Virchow?, *The Lancet*, Vol. 357, 2001
• C.N. Tymchuk et al., Evidence of an inhibitory effect of diet and exercise on prostate cancer cell growth, *Journal of Urology*, September 2001
• Wiygul JB, et al, Supplement Use Among Men With Prostate Cancer, *Urology*, Vol. 66, No. 1, 2005
• Sonn GA, et al, Impact of Diet on Prostate Cancer: A Review. *Prostate Cancer and Prostatic Disease*: Vol. 8, 2005
• Giugliano D and Esposito K, Mediterranean Diet and Cardiovascular Health. *Annals of the New York Academy of Science*, Vol. 1056, 2005

RESOURCES

American Cancer Society
1-800-ACS-2345 (1-800-227-2345)
www.cancer.org

American Urological Association Foundation (AUAF)
410-689-3990
1-866-RING-AUA (1-866-746-4282)
www.auafoundation.org
The AUA Foundation is the nation's leading urologic health
charity that promotes research, education and advocacy. AUA
Foundation's mission is to improve prevention, detection,
treatment and ultimately, cure urologic diseases.

CancerCare
212-712-8400
1-800-813-HOPE (1-800-813-4673)
www.cancercare.org
CancerCare is a national nonprofit organization that provides
free, professional support services to anyone affected by cancer:
people with cancer, caregivers, children, loved ones, and the
bereaved.

Livestrong Foundation
1-877-236-8820
The Livestrong Foundation works to identify the issues faced by
cancer survivors in order to comprehensively improve quality of
life for members of the global cancer community.

National Cancer Institute (NCI)
1-800-4-CANCER (1-800-422-6237)
www.cancer.gov
The National Cancer Institute's Web site (www.cancer.gov)
provides accurate, up-to-date information about many types of
cancer, information about clinical trials, resources for people
dealing with cancer, and information for researchers and health
professionals.

National Prostate Cancer Coalition (NPCC)
202-463-9455
1-888-245-9455
www.fightprostatecancer.org
The National Prostate Cancer Coalition (NPCC) is the largest
advocacy organization dedicated to ending the devastating
impact of prostate cancer on men and their families through
awareness, outreach and advocacy.

Prostate Cancer Foundation (PCF)
310-570-4700
1-800-757-CURE (1-800-757-2873)
www.pcf.org
The Prostate Cancer Foundation (PCF) is the world's largest
philanthropic source of support for prostate cancer research to
discover better treatments and a cure for recurrent prostate
cancer.

Prostate.Net
www.prostate.net
Prostate.net is a website for men who want to get healthy, stay
healthy and lead a life of maximum wellness. Prostate.net's
mission is to massively reduce the millions of cases of prostate
and other men's health disorders diagnosed every year
worldwide.

Us TOO International Prostate Cancer Education & Support
Network
630-795-1002
1-800-80-UsTOO (1-800-808-7866)
www.ustoo.org
This nonprofit organization provides prostate cancer survivors
and their families emotional and educational support through
an international network of local support groups.

ABOUT THE AUTHOR

Steve Vogel is an award-winning copywriter, journalist and author. Over a 25-year career as a freelance writer, he has worked as magazine columnist, sports and features writer, contributing editor and stringer for local and national publications, both online and print.

Published in a half-dozen languages, Steve has won numerous ADDY awards as a copywriter for many of the biggest names in the Fortune 2000 corporate communications world: IBM, Dole Foods, Pratt-Whitney, Tyco, Citrix, among others. Steve is also the recipient of the Hemingway Award for short fiction.

Steve lives in Delray Beach, Florida, with his wife, Lorraine, and son, Nick, when he is home from attending the University of Florida, also Steve's alma mater. He continues to work as a freelance writer, amateur sports photographer and blogger. Steve is currently writing his fourth novel for publication. The other three attempts are still in the drawer.

Book website:
http://www.TheProstateStorm.com
Blog:
http://theprostatestorm.blogspot.com
Facebook:
http://www.facebook.com/TheProstateStorm

www.ingramcontent.com/pod-product-compliance
Lightning Source LLC
Chambersburg PA
CBHW050132280326
41933CB00010B/1347